Surgical Management of Benign Lung Disease

Editors

STEPHEN R. HAZELRIGG
TRAVES D. CRABTREE

THORACIC SURGERY CLINICS

www.thoracic.theclinics.com

Consulting Editor
VIRGINIA R. LITLE

May 2021 • Volume 31 • Number 2

ELSEVIER

1600 John F. Kennedy Boulevard • Suite 1800 • Philadelphia, Pennsylvania, 19103-2899

http://www.thoracic.theclinics.com

THORACIC SURGERY CLINICS Volume 31, Number 2
May 2021 ISSN 1547-4127, ISBN-13: 978-0-323-79345-2

Editor: John Vassallo (j.vassallo@elsevier.com)
Developmental Editor: Jessica Nicole B. Cañaberal

Thoracic Surgery Clinics (ISSN 1547-4127) is published quarterly by Elsevier Inc., 360 Park Avenue South, New York, NY 10010-1710. Months of publication are February, May, August, and November. Business and editorial offices: 1600 John F. Kennedy Boulevard, Suite 1800, Philadelphia, PA 19103-2899. Periodicals postage paid at New York, NY, and additional mailing offices. Subscription prices are $397.00 per year (US individuals), $858.00 per year (US institutions), $100.00 per year (US students), $464.00 per year (Canadian individuals), $888.00 per year (Canadian institutions), $100.00 per year (Canadian students), $225.00 per year (international students), $485.00 per year (international individuals), and $888.00 per year (international institutions). Foreign air speed delivery is included in all Clinics' subscription prices. All prices are subject to change without notice. **POSTMASTER:** Send address changes to Thoracic Surgery Clinics, Elsevier Health Sciences Division, Subscription Customer Service, 3251 Riverport Lane, Maryland Heights, MO 63043. **Customer Service (orders, claims, online, change of address): Telephone: 1-800-654-2452 (U.S. and Canada); 314-447-8871 (outside U.S. and Canada). Fax: 314-447-8029. E-mail: journalscustomerservice-usa@elsevier.com (for print support); journalsonlinesupport-usa@elsevier.com (for online support).**

Reprints. For copies of 100 or more, of articles in this publication, please contact Commercial Rights Department, Elsevier Inc., 360 Park Avenue South, New York, NY 10010-1710. Tel: 212-633-3874; Fax: 212-633-3820; E-mail: reprints@elsevier.com.

Thoracic Surgery Clinics is covered in *MEDLINE/PubMed (Index Medicus), EMBASE/Excerpta Medica, Science Citation Index Expanded (SciSearch®), Journal Citation Reports/Science Edition,* and *Current Contents®/Clinical Medicine.*

Printed in the United States of America.

Contributors

CONSULTING EDITOR

VIRGINIA R. LITLE, MD
Professor, Department of Surgery, Chief,
Division of Thoracic Surgery, Boston
University, Boston, Massachusetts, USA

EDITORS

STEPHEN R. HAZELRIGG, MD
Professor and Former Chairman, SIU
Healthcare, Division of Cardiothoracic Surgery,
Department of Surgery, SIU School of
Medicine, Springfield, Illinois, USA

TRAVES D. CRABTREE, MD
Professor and Chairman, SIU HealthCare,
Division of Cardiothoracic Surgery,
Department of Surgery, SIU School of
Medicine, Springfield, Illinois, USA

AUTHORS

CLAUDIO CAVIEZEL, MD
Senior Surgeon, Department of Thoracic
Surgery, University Hospital Zürich, Zürich,
Switzerland

ROBERT J. CERFOLIO, MD, MBA
Department of Cardiothoracic Surgery, NYU
Langone Health, New York, New York, USA

LAURENS J. CEULEMANS, MD, PhD
Professor of Surgery, Thoracic Surgeon,
Department of Thoracic Surgery, University
Hospitals Leuven, Leuven, Belgium

STEPHANIE H. CHANG, MD
Department of Cardiothoracic Surgery, NYU
Langone Health, New York, New York, USA

TRAVES D. CRABTREE, MD
Professor and Chairman, SIU HealthCare,
Division of Cardiothoracic Surgery,
Department of Surgery, SIU School of
Medicine, Springfield, Illinois, USA

MALCOLM M. DeCAMP, MD
Division of Cardiothoracic Surgery,
Department of Surgery, University of
Wisconsin-Madison, Madison, Wisconsin, USA

NATHALIE FORAY, DO, MS
Department of Internal Medicine, Division of
Pulmonary and Critical Care Medicine, SIU
School of Medicine, Springfield, Illinois, USA

TRAVIS C. GERACI, MD
Department of Cardiothoracic Surgery, NYU
Langone Health, New York, New York, USA

MARK E. GINSBURG, MD
Department of Thoracic Surgery, NewYork-
Presbyterian Columbia University Irving
Medical Center, New York, New York, USA

STEPHEN R. HAZELRIGG, MD
Professor and Former Chairman, SIU
Healthcare, Division of Cardiothoracic Surgery,
Department of Surgery, SIU School of
Medicine, Springfield, Illinois, USA

JOHN HOWINGTON, MD
Professor, Chair of Thoracic Surgery,
Department of Clinical Medicine Education,
University of Tennessee Health Sciences
Center, Ascension Saint Thomas Health,
Nashville, Tennessee, USA

AMIE KENT, MD
Department of Cardiothoracic Surgery, NYU Langone Health, New York, New York, USA

SETH KRANTZ, MD
Chief, Division of Thoracic Surgery, Northshore University HealthSystem, Evanston, Illinois, USA; Clinical Assistant Professor of Surgery, University of Chicago Medicine and Biological Sciences, Chicago, Illinois, USA

NICHOLAS LANZOTTI, MPH
Division of Cardiothoracic Surgery, Department of Surgery, SIU School of Medicine, Springfield, Illinois, USA

PHILIPPE H. LEMAITRE, MD, PhD
Department of Thoracic Surgery, NewYork-Presbyterian Columbia University Irving Medical Center, New York, New York, USA

STEPHEN MARKWELL, MA
Division of Cardiothoracic Surgery, Department of Surgery, SIU School of Medicine, Springfield, Illinois, USA

DANIEL P. McCARTHY, MD, MBA, MEM
Division of Cardiothoracic Surgery, Department of Surgery, University of Wisconsin-Madison, Madison, Wisconsin, USA

KYLE McCULLOUGH, MD
Division of Cardiothoracic Surgery, Department of Surgery, SIU School of Medicine, Springfield, Illinois, USA

ROBERT J. McKENNA Jr, MD
Department of Surgery, John Wayne Cancer Institute, Los Angeles, California, USA; Professor, Thoracic Surgery, Stanford University

BRYAN MEYERS, MD, MPH
Professor of Surgery, Washington University School of Medicine, Barnes-Jewish Hospital, Saint Louis, Missouri, USA

KEITH S. NAUNHEIM, MD
Professor of Surgery, Division of Cardiothoracic Surgery, Saint Louis University School of Medicine, Saint Louis, Missouri, USA

ISABELLE OPITZ, MD
Professor of Surgery, Director of Thoracic Surgery, Department of Thoracic Surgery, University Hospital Zürich, Zürich, Switzerland

JOSEPH J. PLATZ, MD
Assistant Professor of Surgery, Division of Cardiothoracic Surgery, Saint Louis University School of Medicine, Saint Louis, Missouri, USA

SIMRAN RANDHAWA, MD
Washington University School of Medicine, Barnes-Jewish Hospital, Saint Louis, Missouri, USA

NISHA RIZVI, PhD
Division of Cardiothoracic Surgery, Department of Surgery, Center for Clinical Research, SIU School of Medicine, Springfield, Illinois, USA

NICOLAS ROCHE, MD, PhD, FERS
Respiratory Medicine, Pneumologie et Soins Intensifs Respiratoires, APHP Centre, Cochin Hospital, Université de Paris (Descartes), Institut Cochin (UMR 1016), Paris, France

JUSTIN SAWYER, BS
Division of Cardiothoracic Surgery, Department of Surgery, SIU School of Medicine, Springfield, Illinois, USA

DIDIER SCHNEITER, MD
Senior Surgeon, Department of Thoracic Surgery, University Hospital Zürich, Zürich, Switzerland

BENJAMIN SEADLER, BS
Division of Cardiothoracic Surgery, Department of Surgery, SIU School of Medicine, Springfield, Illinois, USA

SAVAN K. SHAH, BS
NYU School of Medicine, NYU Langone Health, New York, New York, USA

JOSHUA R. SONETT, MD
Department of Thoracic Surgery, NewYork-Presbyterian Columbia University Irving Medical Center, New York, New York, USA

BRYAN PAYNE STANIFER, MD, MPH
Department of Thoracic Surgery, NewYork-Presbyterian Columbia University Irving Medical Center, New York, New York, USA

TAYLOR STONE, MD
Department of Internal Medicine, Division of Pulmonary and Critical Care Medicine, SIU School of Medicine, Springfield, Illinois, USA

LAUREN J. TAYLOR, MD
Division of Cardiothoracic Surgery, University
of Colorado, Anschutz Medical Campus,
Aurora, Colorado, USA

SOWMYANARAYANAN THUPPAL, MD, PhD
Division of Cardiothoracic Surgery,
Department of Surgery, Center for Clinical
Research, SIU School of Medicine, Springfield,
Illinois, USA

JANANI VIGNESWARAN, MD, MPH
General Surgery Resident, Department of
Surgery, University of Chicago Medicine and
Biological Sciences, Chicago, Illinois, USA

BRADLEY VOST, BS
Division of Cardiothoracic Surgery,
Department of Surgery, SIU School of
Medicine, Springfield, Illinois, USA

WALTER WEDER, MD
Professor of Surgery, Thoracic Surgeon,
Thoracic Surgery, Thoraxchirurgie Bethanien,
Zürich, Switzerland

PETER WHITE, MD
Department of Internal Medicine, Division of
Pulmonary and Critical Care Medicine, SIU
School of Medicine, Springfield, Illinois, USA

SEAN C. WIGHTMAN, MD
Division of Thoracic Surgery, Keck School of
Medicine of USC, University of Southern
California, Los Angeles, California, USA

Contents

Foreword: Far from Benign: Thoracic Management of Emphysema   xiii

Virginia R. Litle

Preface: Treatment of End-Stage Emphysema   xv

Stephen R. Hazelrigg and Traves D. Crabtree

Systemic Medications in Chronic Obstructive Pulmonary Disease: Use and Outcomes   97

Nicolas Roche

Inhaled therapy remains the cornerstone of chronic obstructive pulmonary disease pharmacologic care, but some systemic treatments can be of help when the burden of the disease remains high. Azithromycin, phosphodiesterase-4 inhibitors, and mucoactive agents can be used in such situations. The major difficulty remains in the identification of the optimal target populations. Another difficulty is to determine how these treatments should be positioned in the global treatment algorithm. For instance, should they be prescribed in addition to other antiinflammatory agents or should they replace them in some cases? Research is ongoing to identify new therapeutic targets.

Critical Analysis of the National Emphysema Treatment Trial Results for Lung-Volume-Reduction Surgery   107

Joseph J. Platz and Keith S. Naunheim

The National Emphysema Treatment Trial compared medical treatment of severe pulmonary emphysema with lung-volume-reduction surgery in a multiinstitutional randomized prospective fashion. Two decades later, this trial remains one of the key sources of information we have on the treatment of advanced emphysematous lung disease. The trial demonstrated the short- and long-term effectiveness of surgical intervention as well as the need for strict patient selection and preoperative workup. Despite these findings, the key failure of the trial was an inability to convince the medical community of the value of surgical resection in the treatment of advanced emphysema.

Analysis of Recent Literature on Lung Volume Reduction Surgery   119

Daniel P. McCarthy, Lauren J. Taylor, and Malcolm M. DeCamp

Publication of the National Emphysema Treatment Trial (NETT) in 2003 established lung volume reduction surgery (LVRS) as a viable treatment of select patients with moderate to severe emphysema, and the only intervention since the availability of ambulatory supplemental oxygen to improve survival. Despite these findings, surgical treatment has been underused in part because of concern for high morbidity and mortality. This article reviews recent literature generated since the original NETT publication, focusing on physiologic implications of LVRS, recent data regarding the safety and durability of LVRS, and patient selection and extension of NETT criteria to other patient populations.

As palliative treatment, lung volume reduction surgery can be offered to a selected subset of chronic obstructive pulmonary disease patients. Careful adherence to established inclusion and exclusion criteria is critical to achieve good outcomes. The evolution of surgical techniques toward minimally invasive approaches has improved outcomes. The fully extrathoracic access combining a subxiphoid incision with subcostal port placement allowed a further decrease in perioperative pain, which favors spontaneous respiratory drive and early postoperative mobilization. Less aggressive resections and better match for size of the hemithorax have contributed to a short-term reduction in morbidity and continued improvements in cardio-pulmonary function.

Chronic obstructive pulmonary usually is subcategorized into 2 groups: chronic bronchitis and emphysema. The main cause of chronic bronchitis and emphysema is smoking; however, alpha1-antitrypsin also has been seen to cause emphysema in patients who are deficient. As symptoms and lung function decline, treatment modalities, such as lung volume reduction surgery, have been used in individuals with chronic obstructive pulmonary disease and upper lobe predominant emphysema. This article analyzes multiple published series where lung volume reduction surgery has been used in individuals with alpha1-antitrypsin deficiency and their overall outcomes.

Postoperative air leak is one of the most common complications after pulmonary resection and contributes to postoperative pain, complications, and increased hospital length of stay. Several risk factors, including both patient and surgical characteristics, increase the frequency of air leaks. Appropriate intraoperative tissue handling is the most important surgical technique to reduce air leaks. Digital drainage systems have improved the management of postoperative air leak via objective data, portability, and ease of use in the outpatient setting. Several treatment strategies have been used to address prolonged air leak, including pleurodesis, blood patch, placement of endobronchial valves, and reoperative surgery.

Lung volume reduction surgery can significantly improve quality of life for properly selected patients who are symptomatic despite maximal medical management for emphysema. This requires a well-constructed multidisciplinary team (including transplant) to evaluate and treat these patients.

Lung volume reduction surgery (LVRS) patient selection guidelines are based on the National Emphysema Treatment Trial. Because of increased mortality and poor improvement in functional outcomes, patients with non–upper lobe emphysema and low baseline exercise capacity are determined as poor candidates for LVRS. In well-selected patients with heterogeneous emphysema, LVRS has a durable long-term outcome at up to 5-years of follow-up. Five-year survival rates in patients range between 63% and 78%. LVRS seems a durable alternative for end-stage heterogeneous emphysema in patients not eligible for lung transplantation. Future studies will help identify eligible patients with homogeneous emphysema for LVRS.

Endobronchial valve therapy has evolved over the past decade, with demonstration of significant improvements in pulmonary function, 6-minute walk distance, and quality of life in patients with end-stage chronic obstructive lung disease. Appropriate patient selection is crucial, with identification of the most diseased lobe and of a target lobe with minimal to no collateral ventilation. Endobronchial valve therapy typically is utilized in patients with heterogeneous disease but may be indicated in select patients with homogeneous disease. Morbidity and mortality have been lower than historically reported with lung volume reduction surgery, but complications related to pneumothoraces remain a challenge.

Randomized controlled trials have demonstrated that lung volume reduction surgery (LVRS) improves exercise capacity, lung function, and quality of life in patients with heterogenous emphysema on computed tomographic and perfusion scan. However, most patients have a nonheterogenous type of destruction. These patients, summarized under "homogeneous emphysema," may also benefit from LVRS as long they are severely hyperinflated, and adequate function is remaining with a diffusing capacity of the lungs for carbon monoxide greater than 20% and no pulmonary hypertension. Surgical mortality is low when patients are well selected.

Chronic obstructive pulmonary disease is a challenging disease to treat, and at advanced stages of the disease, procedural interventions become some of the only effective methods for improving quality of life. However, these procedures are often very costly. This article reviews the medical literature on cost-effectiveness of lung volume reduction surgery and bronchoscopic valve placement for lung volume reduction. It discusses the anticipated costs and economic impact in the future as technique is perfected and outcomes are improved.

Although there are multiple pharmacologic and nonpharmacological options to alleviate symptoms of emphysema, none of these treatment modalities halts disease progression. The expanding disease burden has led to development of innovative therapeutic strategies that also aim to induce lung volume reduction. Bronchoscopic lung volume reduction originated in 2001 and has continued to grow rapidly ever since. This article discusses more recent developments in bronchoscopic and novel interventions and speculates on how these novel strategies may impact the future of lung reduction interventions.

THORACIC SURGERY CLINICS

SERIES OF RELATED INTEREST

Surgical Clinics
http://www.surgical.theclinics.com

Surgical Oncology Clinics
http://www.surgonc.theclinics.com

Advances in Surgery
http://www.advancessurgery.com

THE CLINICS ARE AVAILABLE ONLINE!
Access your subscription at:
www.theclinics.com

Foreword
Far from Benign: Thoracic Management of Emphysema

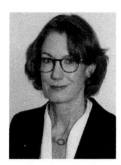

Virginia R. Litle, MD
Consulting Editor

We are excited to bring you this focused issue for the *Thoracic Surgery Clinics* on "Surgical Management of Benign Lung Disease." As per the Preface title by guest editors Hazelrigg and Crabtree, this is more specifically a treatise on End-Stage Emphysema. The contributing authors focused on interventional approaches to improving the quality of life of patients with emphysema, a costly and deadly disease impacting over 3 million Americans. This emphysema issue is about reduction and not replacement, that refers to lung transplant, which we will read about in next year's issue to be guest edited by Drs Kukreja and Venado. From maximally invasive lung volume reduction surgery (LVRS) via sternotomy to least-invasive approaches with endobronchial valves, the management continues to evolve. It wasn't that long ago that many of us cared for the challenging patients with prolonged air leaks after their LVRS surgery. The medical community didn't necessarily see this, yet they have focused on the dated mortalities of the procedures and subsequently have failed to appreciate the benefits derived from careful selection of patients. As McCarthy and colleagues write: "Recent data demonstrate that LVRS may be performed safely with 6-month mortality as low as 0% to 1.5% and durable functional improvements." The recurring theme in these submissions is that we could be doing more to help these patients with end-stage lung disease and emphysema. The lack of interventions perhaps may be impacted by the smoking stigma associated with lung cancer.

Advanced emphysematous lung disease is a major public health problem and a burden on our health care system. Take-home messages from this issue include the following: (1) convince the medical community that in the twenty-first century there is a role for interventional therapies for emphysema; and (2) multidisciplinary conferences for end-stage lung disease should be as common as tumor boards. Not all clinicians have the luxury of an institutional lung transplant program, but they all know how to pick up the phone and make a referral.

Thank you to our contributors and to guest editors, Drs Hazelrigg and Crabtree, for providing a thorough compendium of clinically relevant evidence to advance this area of medicine. Please share it with our pulmonary and medical colleagues!

Sincerely,

Virginia R. Litle, MD
Division of Thoracic Surgery
Department of Surgery
Boston University
88 East Newton Street
Collamore Building, Suite 7380
Boston, MA 02118, USA

E-mail address:
Virginia.litle@bmc.org

Twitter: @vlitlemd (V.R. Litle)

Thorac Surg Clin 31 (2021) xiii
https://doi.org/10.1016/j.thorsurg.2021.03.001
1547-4127/21/© 2021 Published by Elsevier Inc.

Preface
Treatment of End-Stage Emphysema

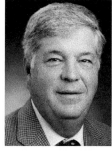
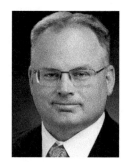

Stephen R. Hazelrigg, MD   Traves D. Crabtree, MD

Editors

Surgical management of end-stage emphysema has been and continues to be both interesting and ever changing. The modern-day surgical treatment began in the early 1990s using laser techniques to try to cause some volume reduction. This was followed by more effective stapled resection of the emphysematous areas and better understanding of proper patient selection. More recently, we have seen the introduction of endobronchial valves and other novel treatments trying to achieve results less invasively. This issue of *Thoracic Surgery Clinics* attempts to provide the most current data available and opinions on surgical options and the most appropriate treatments.

The most recent and up-to-date literature is provided in this issue, and it includes discussions on outcomes as well as indications for lung volume reduction surgery, endobronchial valves, and other novel treatments. Economic considerations are explored, and we attempt to provide a glimpse into what our experts see in the future for the treatment of emphysema.

Areas such as how best to treat emphysema patients with the various options, particularly trying to decide between lung volume reduction surgery and endobronchial valves, are continually evolving. Having a cohesive and comprehensive multidisciplinary program that offers all the options would appear to be an important step in providing the best treatment.

I think this issue provides a comprehensive review for those interested in the topic of emphysema and the options for intervention. I trust it will be both educational and entertaining.

I am very appreciative of all the authors for their contributions to this issue of *Thoracic Surgery Clinics*.

It is not hard to imagine that this area will see a large increase in both interest and treatment in the future.

Stephen R. Hazelrigg, MD
SIU Healthcare
Division of Cardiothoracic Surgery
Department of Surgery
701 North First Street
PO Box 19679
Springfield, IL 62794-9679, USA

Traves D. Crabtree, MD
SIU HealthCare
Division of Cardiothoracic Surgery
Department of Surgery
701 North First Street
PO Box 19679
Springfield, IL 62794-9679, USA

E-mail addresses:
shazelrigg@siumed.edu (S.R. Hazelrigg)
tcrabtree53@siumed.edu (T.D. Crabtree)

Thorac Surg Clin 31 (2021) xv
https://doi.org/10.1016/j.thorsurg.2021.02.009
1547-4127/21/© 2021 Published by Elsevier Inc.

Systemic Medications in Chronic Obstructive Pulmonary Disease
Use and Outcomes

Nicolas Roche, MD, PhD, FERS

KEYWORDS

- COPD • Theophylline • Phosphodiesterase inhibitors • Oral corticosteroids • Macrolides
- Mucoactive agents • Alpha1-antitrypsin • Morphine

KEY POINTS

- Systemic treatments of chronic obstructive pulmonary disease (COPD) are not first-line therapeutic options.
- The benefit/risk ratio of oral beta2-adrenergic agonists and xanthines is not favorable.
- Azithromycin, phosphodiesterase 4 inhibitors, and mucomodifiers can contribute to exacerbation prevention in patients on inhaled therapy.
- The long-term use of systemic corticosteroids in COPD should be strongly discouraged.
- Several biologics are currently in development for COPD therapy and may prove useful in particular subpopulations identified through the use of specific biomarkers.

INTRODUCTION

Chronic obstructive pulmonary disease (COPD) is now defined by the coexistence of chronic respiratory symptoms and permanent (ie, not fully reversible) airflow limitation, caused by airways and parenchymal disease.[1] The development of airflow obstruction and emphysema is the consequence of a close interplay between inflammation, innate and adaptive immune reactions, protease-antiprotease imbalance, and oxidative stress, leading to airway wall and parenchymal remodeling and mucus hypersecretion.[2–6] Associated phenomena include chronic infection/colonization/microbiota modifications, autoimmunity, senescence, and systemic inflammation.[7,8]

Although some decades ago systemic treatments (ie, theophylline and oral corticosteroids for very severe cases) represented the main therapeutic approach for patients with COPD, inhaled medications are now the cornerstone of COPD treatment.[1] They have the obvious advantage of delivering high local concentrations of effective medication, while minimizing systemic absorption and side effects. However, because of these properties, they do not exert any significant effect on the systemic components of the disease, which have been repeatedly emphasized in the last 15 years.[9] The comorbidities and systemic features frequently seen in patients with COPD include muscle deconditioning, malnutrition, osteoporosis, psychological distress (anxiety-depression), cognitive impairment, metabolic and cardiovascular diseases, anemia, and lung cancer.[10–12] In the mid 2000s there was great enthusiasm around the concept of systemic inflammation as a common trigger for all of these conditions, with many studies showing increases in several systemic inflammatory biomarkers.

This article originally appeared in *Clinics in Chest Medicine*, Volume 41, Issue 3, September 2020.

Dr N. Roche reports grants and personal fees from Boehringer Ingelheim, Novartis, and Pfizer, and personal fees from Teva, GSK, AstraZeneca, Chiesi, Mundipharma, Cipla, Sanofi, Sandoz, 3M, Trudell, and Zambon.

Respiratory Medicine, Pneumologie et Soins Intensifs Respiratoires, APHP Centre, Cochin Hospital, Université de Paris (Descartes), Institut Cochin (UMR 1016), 27, rue du Fbg St Jacques, Paris 75014, France

E-mail address: nicolas.roche@aphp.fr

However, the exact relation between COPD and underlying pathophysiologic mechanisms remained uncertain. At present, decreased physical activity (also associated with systemic inflammation) is viewed as a major common contributor to most systemic aspects of COPD.[13] The increased frequency of cardiovascular events and treatments in patients with COPD also led to some interest in the possible interaction between inflammatory bursts and/or increases in lung hyperinflation with COPD outcomes, and this is the most plausible mechanism helping explain the increased risk of major cardiovascular events following acute exacerbations.[10]

In addition to their lack of effects on the systemic component of COPD, inhaled treatments may not be sufficiently effective to deliver pharmaceutical agents to the small airways, where most of the disease processes outlined earlier reside.[14]

This article reviews the effects of systemic agents with a main focus on clinical outcomes and long-term maintenance use. Pharmaceutical families of interest include oral beta2 agonists, theophylline, phosphodiesterase (PDE) inhibitors, macrolides with antiinflammatory properties and other antibiotics, mucoactive agents, corticosteroids, antileukotrienes, cardiovascular drugs, and biologics.

ORAL BETA2-ADRENERGIC AGONISTS

The benefit/risk ratio of oral beta2 agonists is much less favorable than that of their inhaled counterparts, because high systemic levels are required to achieve sufficient local concentrations leading to bronchodilation. At therapeutic doses, side effects (tremor, tachycardia) are more frequent and intense, whereas bronchodilation is similar[15] or less pronounced[16] than the inhaled presentation. In addition, these agents have been assessed only in small short-term studies with no patient-reported outcome end points. As a consequence, they are not recommended for COPD treatment except when the use of any inhaled treatment is impossible.

XANTHINES, THEOPHYLLINE

Theophylline is a xanthine structurally similar to caffeine that was initially developed for asthma in the late 1930s, at a time when COPD was not even well recognized.[17–19] Its main mechanisms of action are adenosine receptor (A1 and A2) inhibition (high potency at therapeutic concentrations) and (weak) PDE-3 and PDE-4 selective inhibition at higher and poorly tolerated concentrations.[20] Through these pathways, it exerts numerous immunomodulatory and antiinflammatory effects and has weak bronchodilator properties. Interestingly, theophylline decreases neutrophilic and eosinophilic airways inflammation, which can both be involved in patients with COPD, depending on the underlying endotype (ie, pathophysiologic profile). It also modulates lymphocytes functions.

The acute physiologic effects of theophylline include bronchodilation, lung deflation, improved gas exchanges, increased diaphragmatic function, reduced work of breathing, and improved mucociliary clearance. How these numerous demonstrable effects translate into clinical improvements is less clear, which is largely explained by the narrow therapeutic index of the drug; for instance, bronchodilation and diaphragmatic improvements need high doses to be clinically meaningful, which exposes patients to risks of serious dose/concentration-dependent side effects such as gastrointestinal (GI) perturbations (nausea, vomiting, exacerbated gastroesophageal reflux), tremor, sleep disturbance, headache, seizures, arrhythmias, and heart failure. In addition, many factors can interact with theophylline serum concentrations, including diseases that are frequently seen in patients with COPD, such as heart failure, liver disease, and smoking. In addition, theophylline serum concentrations vary depending on its interaction with several concomitant drugs (including antibiotics used in COPD exacerbations), the elimination of which is modulated by the cytochrome P (CYP) 1A2 or CYP3A4 coenzymatic activity (**Table 1**). Thus, using theophylline often requires monitoring its blood concentrations, further influencing its ease of use. As a consequence, and particularly in acute situations, the acute use of theophylline has been widely abandoned because of the need for high serum concentrations to achieve clinically meaningful bronchodilation or diaphragmatic improvement, and the associated risk of significant toxicity.

Regarding long-term use, there has been some interest in one particular property of theophylline: restoration of histone-deacetylase 2 (HDAC2) activity.[21] HDAC2 is an important cofactor of corticosteroids effects because it interacts with the corticosteroid-glucocorticoid receptor, contributing to chromatin condensation and thereby inhibiting the transcription and subsequent expression of proinflammatory genes (transrepression).[22] In smokers, and even more in patients with COPD, the oxidative stress impairs HDAC2 function, representing 1 of the numerous mechanisms of corticosteroid resistance.[23] Thus, conceptually theophylline could restore the effects of corticosteroids, which are reduced in smokers and in COPD. This mode of action could be of

Table 1
Main modulators of theophylline's pharmacokinetics

Effect	Increased Bioavailability	Reduced Bioavailability
Disease/condition	Viral infections Congestive heart failure Liver diseases	—
Age	—	Children<16 y
Toxic agents	—	Cigarette and marijuana smoking
Medications (through CYP1A2 and CYP3A4 modulation)	Erythromycin, clarithromycin (not azithromycin), ciprofloxacin (not ofloxacin), cimetidine (not ranitidine) allopurinol, serotonin uptake inhibitors, flu vaccination	Phenytoin, phenobarbitone, rifampicin

Data from Refs.[18,20]

particular interest because it occurs at serum concentrations that are approximately half the threshold of toxicity. Following encouraging results from in vitro experiments on HDAC2 activity and corticosteroid cellular effects, this hypothesis has been clinically tested in 2 randomized controlled trials, with disappointing results regarding all variables of clinical interest (ie, lung function, exacerbations, symptoms, and quality of life).[24,25]

As a consequence, the use of theophylline has been largely abandoned as part of long-term maintenance therapy. However, in some areas of the world, Cost-issues are such that theophylline is one of a few affordable options, together with a few low-cost (but still very effective) inhaled drugs such as salbutamol and beclomethasone.

The theophylline/xanthines family includes not only theophylline but also its derivatives aminophylline (the oldest one), bamiphylline, and doxophylline. The main potential difference between these agents is the efficacy/safety profile, which might be better for doxophylline according to a recent network meta-analysis.[19] How this translates into clinical superiority at the individual patient level is not fully clear.

PHOSPHODIESTERASE 4 INHIBITORS

PDE-4 inhibitors are often wrongly considered as modern theophyllines. This concept is not valid because most of the clinical effect of theophylline observed at nontoxic doses are linked to adenosine receptor antagonism, whereas effective PDE inhibition occurs only at toxic or close-to-toxic doses. Real selective PDE inhibitors commercially available at present are limited to one agent, roflumilast, which is not authorized or reimbursed in all countries. Another agent,

cilomilast, was provisionally approved in the early 2000s but its development has been abandoned because of concerns about its efficacy/safety profile.[26]

There are many subtypes of PDE-4 (A, B, C, and D) and more than 25 isoforms, many of which are expressed in various inflammatory and resident cell types in the airways.[17,27,28] The potential beneficial effects of PDE-4 inhibition are numerous because PDE-4 is involved in cyclic AMP (cAMP) degradation. Thus, PDE-4 inhibition increases cellular levels of cAMP, which acts as an antiinflammatory second messenger decreasing the release of inflammatory mediators and the expression of proinflammatory surface receptors (eg, adhesion molecules) by neutrophils and other cell types, including macrophages, eosinophils, and T lymphocytes. Roflumilast (through its active metabolite roflumilast N-oxide) reduces the recruitment of inflammatory cells in the airways. cAMP is also involved in smooth muscle relaxation, but the bronchodilator effect of roflumilast at therapeutic concentrations is limited. In animal models, roflumilast prevents cigarette smoke–induced lung inflammation and emphysema.[18]

In humans, following the first studies and their subgroup analyses, roflumilast has been shown to reduce the risk of exacerbations in patients with COPD and frequent exacerbations (or previous hospitalization), severe airflow obstruction (Global initiative on Obstructive Lung Disease [GOLD] 3–4, postbronchodilator forced expiratory volume in 1 second [FEV_1] <50% predicted), symptoms of chronic bronchitis, and receiving bronchodilator therapy.[29] This beneficial effect occurs even in patients receiving concomitant treatment with inhaled long-acting bronchodilators and corticosteroids and is accompanied by an improvement in lung function, although the increase in FEV$_1$ (mean, 51 mL) does not reach the classic (but debatable for therapies administered on top of active medications) threshold for clinical significance (100 mL).[30] These effects have been confirmed by Cochrane systematic reviews collating data from 20 studies using roflumilast in more than 17,000 participants,[29] in which small improvements in symptoms and quality of life were also noted.

Roflumilast shares GI side effects with xanthines but, in contrast with those agents, it is not associated with an increased risk of cardiovascular effects. It can induce moderate weight loss (3 kg on average), mostly related to a decrease in fat mass. GI side effects can lead to treatment interruption.

Compounds with both PDE-3 and PDE-4 inhibitory activity have been assessed in humans with no success because of lack or safety and/or unacceptable side effects. A new agent of this family administered through the inhaled route, ensifentrine, is currently being tested in clinical trials.[31] Currently available data are insufficient to draw conclusions.

MACROLIDES AND OTHER ANTIBIOTICS

The most studied macrolide for long-term maintenance therapy in COPD is azithromycin,[32,33] although earlier clinical studies were reported using erythromycin.[34] Antiinflammatory and immune-modulating properties are a feature of these macrolides.[18,35] Their first applications were the successful treatment of diffuse panbronchiolitis with erythromycin, and cystic fibrosis colonized by *Pseudomonas aeruginosa* with azithromycin. Animal models have confirmed the antiinflammatory effects of this agent, which can also prevent cigarette smoke–induced development of emphysema.[18,35] Macrolides also have the potential to augment HDAC2 expression, thereby potentially restoring corticosteroid sensitivity.

During the late 2000s, 3 studies showed the preventive effect of erythromycin on exacerbation occurrences. Subsequent trials showed a similar effect using azithromycin. Although some individual studies failed to achieve the same success, an overall positive effect was shown in a meta-analysis.[36] Studies with roxithromycin and clarithromycin did not provide convincing evidence but did not have a sufficiently robust design because they had a low sample size and were of limited duration.[35]

Considering the beneficial effect of both erythromycin and azithromycin (although they have never been directly compared), 4 main questions arise.

First, selection of the best agent and the best scheme of administration. In terms of convenience of use, azithromycin is clearly the preferred drug: once versus twice or 3 times a day for erythromycin. Trials used a 250 mg/d or greater than 500 mg 3 times a week scheme,[35] although 250 mg 3 times a week is probably used more often in clinical practice as in cystic fibrosis (in which the efficacy of this protocol was shown), despite a lack of formal evaluation in COPD.

Second, the most appropriate target population. The largest study with erythromycin recruited 109 patients in a single center. There were no exacerbation-related inclusion criteria, but more than one-third of the population reported at least 3 exacerbations during the 12 months preceding inclusion, and median exacerbation frequency in the placebo group was 2, suggesting a population of frequent exacerbators.[37] The rate reduction of exacerbations in the active arm was 36% and, in addition, erythromycin reduced not only the rate but also the duration of exacerbations. Responders analysis was not performed and would have been difficult considering the limited sample size. The effect on exacerbation was not associated with effects on biomarkers of inflammation or bacterial loads in the airways, preventing any firm conclusions regarding the mechanisms of observed efficacy. Azithromycin was studied over 12 months in the largest macrolide trial (n = 1142).[32] Patients were on supplemental oxygen, had received systemic corticosteroids, or had been hospitalized for an exacerbation during the previous year. There was a 17% overall risk reduction in exacerbations. Responders analysis found the greatest benefit in ex-smokers, older patients, and milder GOLD stages.[38] However this analysis was post hoc, requiring further confirmation before drawing firm conclusions. The other 12-month study on azithromycin was performed in patients with a history of 3 or more exacerbations in the previous year, most of whom received triple inhaled therapy. Overall it remains difficult to define a specific target subgroup, although baseline exacerbation risk is an appropriate selection criterion.

The third question relates to risks associated with long-term macrolide therapy.[35] GI side effects (diarrhea), impairments in liver function, and a minimal increase in hearing loss have been reported. Although there is a theoretic risk of increased cardiac arrhythmias, caused by the potential increase in the corrected QT (QTc) electrocardiographic interval, this was not observed in any of the trials. However, patients with prolonged QTc interval were excluded from those trials. In practice, it may be important to consider its use primarily in patients with normal electrocardiograms. An increase in the proportion of macrolide-resistant microorganisms in nasal swabs has been observed, although the absolute number of patients colonized by such bacteria did not change. The bacteriologic consequences of long-term macrolide use in COPD populations remains unknown. The last important question is the duration of treatment. For this question, there is no firm answer at present. Conclusive trials have lasted 6 to 12 months, and no trial of sequential administration (eg, during the winter period) has been performed.

Regarding other (nonmacrolide) antibiotics, the only sufficiently powered trial was performed with pulsed moxifloxacin (400 mg/d 5 days every 8 weeks), which produced a nonsignificant trend toward a reduction in exacerbations and is thus considered a negative trial.[39]

MUCOMODIFIERS

There are 2 main potential reasons for considering the use of mucoactive agents in COPD[40]: first, chronic mucus hypersecretion is thought to play an important role in the pathophysiology and natural course of the disease. The mucus is more abundant and viscous in many patients with COPD and is responsible for small airways obstruction, which is associated with poor prognosis in patients undergoing lung volume reduction surgery. In smokers and patients with COPDs, chronic mucus hypersecretion is also associated with several prognostic variables (FEV_1 decline and development of COPD, exacerbation and hospitalization risk, and mortality). Mucin concentrations (MUC5B, MUC5AC) seem to play a key role in the pathogenesis of chronic bronchitis.[5]

Several mucoactive agents have antioxidant properties, and oxidative stress is thought to be involved in the pathobiology of COPD, both at local (airways) and systemic levels.[6] Its consequences include inflammatory cells recruitment, protease-antiprotease imbalance, and production of proinflammatory mediators. Paradoxically, there has been no firm demonstration of an effect of most mucoactive agents on mucociliary clearance in vivo in humans. In vitro data and animal models found effects on airway wall remodeling, chemotaxis, and activation of neutrophils and monocytes/macrophages as well as decreasing bacterial adherence. In vivo during acute exacerbations, a reduction in levels of inflammatory markers and an improvement in bacterial elimination and symptoms has been found but was not accompanied by effects on hard end points such as lung function or length of stay in the hospital,

questioning the clinical relevance of biological effects. Some mucoactive agents (carbocysteine, N-acetylcysteine, erdosteine, and ambroxol) have reduced the occurrence of COPD exacerbations in several trials, a finding that is supported by the results of a meta-analysis.[41] One of those trials found a reduction in exacerbation rate only in patients not taking inhaled corticosteroids (ICS), whereas the other found a reduction in the overall population, in which only a minority (<20%) of patients received ICS, suggesting that mucoactive agents may prove effective only in patients with suboptimal inhaled therapy. This point was further tested in a specifically designed large study that did not find any interaction between ICS and effects of N-acetylcysteine on exacerbations occurrence. This finding was confirmed in a more recent network meta-analysis in which a metaregression was performed to identify factors associated with treatment response.[41] Surprisingly, this analysis identified a trend toward less response in Chinese populations. This finding needs to be interpreted with caution considering the significant heterogeneity observed in the meta-analysis.

ORAL CORTICOSTEROIDS

The long-term use of oral corticosteroids is discouraged in COPD because of the well-known burden of side effects,[42] contrasting with the lack of evidence of clinically relevant beneficial effects.

Systemic dose-dependent side effects include fractures, diabetes, cataracts, hypertension, open-angle glaucoma, skin bruising, muscular weakness, cardiovascular events, and cerebrovascular events. Many of these effects can have major consequences leading to severe health status impairment. In addition, the use of oral corticosteroids has been linked to increased mortality and reduced efficacy of nutritional supplementation, a component of pulmonary rehabilitation.[43,44] The combination of COPD and oral corticosteroids also increases the risk of infections that may have particularly disastrous consequences in patients with severe lung function impairment, such as mycobacteria, Aspergillus spp, and various types of bacteria involved in chronic airways colonization/infection and pneumonia.

The most recent meta-analysis by the Cochrane Collaboration on oral corticosteroids for stable COPD was published in 2005.[45] Treatment lasted more than 3 weeks in only 5 studies among the 24 that were identified. Combining all studies, the mean FEV_1 improvement was 53 mL, half the minimal clinically important difference. The proportion of FEV_1 responders (>20% increase relative to baseline) was approximately 2.5 times higher with oral steroids than on placebo. Effects were more prominent with higher dosages (>30 mg/d vs 7–15 mg/d), associated with more risks of side effects. Increases in walking distance were statistically significant but not clinically relevant (29 m with the 12-minute walk test), and most of these studies were short term. Some symptomatic and health status differences were reported but considered insignificant from a clinical perspective. Oral corticosteroids did not prevent exacerbations but the studies were not designed to test this end point in a robust manner.

The considerations presented here are valid only for patients with COPD and no associated asthma. The situation may be different in patients with COPD associated with predominating severe asthma, the subject of another article in this issue.

ANTILEUKOTRIENES

Antileukotriene agents are not recommended in COPD.[1] Only very few properly designed studies have been performed to assess their effects in this population. There are 2 types of available agents[18]: 5-lipoxygenase (LO) or 5-LO–activating protein inhibitors and cysteinyl-leukotrienes (Cys-LTs: LT-C4, D4, E4) receptor antagonists. Their purpose is to reduce the production of leukotrienes with proinflammatory activity (LTB4, product of the 5-LO pathway) or to decrease effects on airway smooth muscle, mucus secretion, vascular permeability, and mucociliary clearance (Cys-LTs). In 2015, 7 studies were identified, 3 of which were nonrandomized (2 with montelukast, 1 with zafirlukast). Among the 4 others, 1 dealt with zileuton (for acute exacerbations), 1 with montelukast, and 2 with products that have been secondarily abandoned. All these randomized trials were short term, whereas 2 observational studies (1 prospective, 1 retrospective) had a duration of at least 12 months.[46] Thus, from a review of all of these studies, it is clear that anti-LTs have not been properly assessed in COPD. In only 1 (short-term) randomized controlled trial (RCT) with montelukast, some nonsignificant effects on symptoms (dyspnea, sputum production) and lung function were reported.[46]

CARDIOVASCULAR/METABOLIC TREATMENTS

There is a strong interaction between COPD and cardiovascular diseases, both sharing common risk factors[10]; however, the increased cross-prevalence of these conditions is not explained simply by smoking. As mentioned earlier, this association may relate to systemic inflammation and/or decreased daily physical activity, both of which are interrelated. Impairment of cardiac function caused by lung hyperinflation may also play a role, as well as chronic or intermittent hypoxia. In addition, the burden (eg, in terms of dyspnea and exacerbations) and prognosis of COPD is impaired in the presence of cardiovascular diseases. Reciprocally, there is an increased frequency of COPD in patients with cardiovascular conditions, and COPD impairs their prognosis. Consequently, cardiovascular drugs are frequently used in patients with COPD. In addition, cardiovascular events are more frequent during and after COPD exacerbations, of which they can represent either complications or part of differential diagnoses. Because of these strong interactions, there has been a lot of interest in the potential effects of cardiovascular drugs in patients with COPD.

The first question that was raised related to the safety of β-blockers in patients with COPD: these agents, especially those with poor beta1-adrenoreceptor selectivity, can enhance airway smooth muscle contractions and, thereby worsen airflow limitation, through beta2-adrenoreceptor antagonism. In clinical trials of β-blockers for ischemic heart disease, patients with COPD were found to benefit as much as, or even more than, those with no COPD in terms of survival.[47] The effect of cardioselective β1-blockers on lung function seems very limited, if any, and these agents do not increase the occurrence of respiratory symptoms. In addition, they do not impair respiratory outcomes when continued during acute exacerbations. Observational studies had even suggested that β-blockers could decrease the risk of COPD exacerbations and related hospitalizations and mortality. However, a recent large controlled trial in the United States did not confirm this hypothesis, and found a worse outcome, including risk of death in patients randomized to receive β-blockers and who had no cardiovascular indication of beta1-blockade.[48]

Similarly, retrospective database or prospective cohort studies suggested some benefits from statins in terms of exacerbation risk. Such effects could be explained by the pleiotropic antiinflammatory effects of statins, which could control the systemic inflammation observed in many patients with COPD. However, again a randomized controlled trial did not report any effect on exacerbation rate or mortality in patients with no cardiovascular or metabolic indication.[49]

Renin-angiotensin-aldosterone system inhibitors can have antiinflammatory, antifibrotic, and antioxidant effects that could be of interest in COPD.[10] It has even been suggested that these agents have some potential to prevent emphysema progression.[50] However, no clinical advantage related to the use of these agents has ever been formally established in adequately designed studies.

BIOLOGICS

Inflammation, oxidative stress, and airway and parenchymal remodeling, including fibrosis, all represent potential targets for biologics directed at modulating (upstream or downstream) their mediators, biological triggers, or signaling pathways. Their intimate mechanisms are involved in the clinical manifestations of COPD, including dyspnea and exacerbations, as well as in disease progression. However, this involvement is highly heterogeneous and the disease biology is still incompletely deciphered, making it difficult to identify the most relevant targets and define the corresponding patient populations. Heterogeneity applies not only to stable state but also to exacerbations. In addition, COPD is a slowly evolutive disease with an overall low reactivity to any pharmacologic intervention to date. These properties create additional hurdles when testing new agents clinically. Although clinical phenotypes correspond with clinical features or combinations of features associated with disease progression and/or treatment responses, endotypes are underlying biological mechanisms that can be identified through biomarkers.[51,52] How the disease can be split into phenotypes and endotypes is much less clear in COPD than in asthma.[53] In addition, because there is some marked overlap and discrepancies between phenotypes and between them and endotypes, the current trend is to adopt the concept of individual treatable traits that can be independently targeted by dedicated interventions.[54] Altogether, these traits cover the entire spectrum of asthma, COPD, and complex overlapping/intricate situations. Among them, eosinophilic COPD triggers particular interest.

The central role of systemic and local inflammation in COPD pathophysiology suggested that anti–tumor necrosis factor (THF) agents could have some potential to influence the natural history of the disease. In addition, TNF-alpha has been shown to induce emphysema in animal models. However, clinical trials gave disappointing results, in terms of both effects on markers of local (sputum) and systemic inflammation, and clinical outcomes.[55,56]

More recently, anti–interleukin-5 (IL-5) agents have been tested in COPD. These agents (IL-5 inhibitor or IL-5 receptor blocker) primarily target eosinophilic inflammation. In 2 parallel RCTs using mepolizumab (IL-5 inhibitor), 1 of the trials showed a reduction in the risk of COPD exacerbations (−23%) in patients with higher (>300/µL) blood eosinophil counts (considered as a reliable surrogate for sputum eosinophils).[57] However, these results were not significant in the other study. Further, there was no difference in lung function or health status in either study compared with the placebo arm. The larger and more recent study using benralizumab (IL-5 receptor blocker) did not reduce exacerbation rate in patients with eosinophilic COPD (>220 cells/µL). Therefore, additional data need to be gathered before these treatments can be recommended.

ALPHA1-ANTITRYPSIN AUGMENTATION THERAPY

Because severe alpha1-antitrypsin (AAT) deficiency is a rare disease, RCTs are difficult to conduct. A European Respiratory Society taskforce recently performed a systematic review that identified 8 RCTs and 17 observational studies (11 of which were uncontrolled) assessing the effects of augmentation therapy on various clinical and imaging outcomes.[58] Only 3 RCTs were placebo controlled. There was a beneficial effect on emphysema progression as assessed by computed tomography (CT) scan, but efficacy could not be shown in terms of clinical outcomes. However, such efficacy (although subject to more biases) was suggested by some observational studies. In addition, emphysema progression on CT scan is associated with mortality and quality of life, suggesting that it may represent a clinically relevant outcome. Therefore, several guidelines recommend augmentation therapy in AAT-deficient patients with emphysema and progressive disease.[1]

SYSTEMIC TREATMENTS FOR DYSPNEA

Dyspnea is the most important and relevant symptom of patients with COPD. It is the limiting element of exercise capacity/tolerance and daily activity. Therefore, relieving dyspnea is one of the major goals of COPD care. First-line approaches include bronchodilators and rehabilitation. Interventional techniques such as lung volume reduction can be considered in highly selected patient populations. In some patients, dyspnea remains refractory to those therapies. In such instances, benzodiazepines and morphine have been considered, but they remain seldom prescribed as part of routine practice.[59] In 2016, a Cochrane Review identified 26 RCTs with more than 500 patients with refractory breathlessness in the context of advanced disease and terminal

Table 2
Examples of systemic treatments targeting specific subpopulations/treatable traits in chronic obstructive pulmonary disease

Treatment	Subpopulation/ Treatable Trait
Established	
PDE-4 inhibitors (roflumilast)	Severe airflow obstruction, repeated exacerbations, chronic mucus hyperproduction, on top of long-acting bronchodilators
AAT	AAT deficiency
Putative	
Azithromycin	Ex-smokers, older patients, milder airflow obstruction Airway bacterial colonization/ chronic infection Repeated bacterial exacerbations
Anti–IL-5 agents	Eosinophilic COPD
Mucoactive agents	Chronic mucus hyperproduction

illness. In 14 studies, recruited subjects were primarily or exclusively patients with COPD. Altogether, the quality of evidence was deemed low or very low, but some evidence of dyspnea alleviation was found. In parallel, drowsiness, nausea and vomiting, and constipation were frequent (13%, 20%, and 18%, respectively).[60] Thus, the benefit/risk ratio needs to be carefully considered on an individual basis, balancing the risk of side effects and the burden of dyspnea. In summary, for very breathless patients, a trial can be initiated under close monitoring and stopped if the benefits are not evident or if side effects limit its use.

In a similar way, the last Cochrane Review on benzodiazepines for dyspnea was performed in 2016 and included 8 studies in patients with advanced cancer or COPD, in which benzodiazepines were compared with placebo, promethazine, or morphine. No demonstration of positive effects was found, although the investigators found less drowsiness than with morphine.

SUMMARY

Although numerous systemic treatments for COPD exist, they are positioned late in treatment algorithms, with inhaled therapy remaining the cornerstone of treatment. However, when inhaled therapy is not sufficient to control the burden of disease, oral therapies such as PDE-4 inhibitors, azithromycin, or mucoactive agents can be of help in some patients (**Table 2**), especially to reduce the risk of exacerbations. The major difficulty here is to choose the appropriate responder and how these treatments should be positioned in the global treatment algorithm. For instance, should they be prescribed in addition to other anti-inflammatory agents (ie, corticosteroids) or should they replace them in some specific subgroups of patients? Some currently available biologics used in severe asthma could also be effective in some patient categories (eosinophilic COPD), but additional studies centered on well-selected candidates are needed. Some oral agents, such as beta2-adrenergic agents and particularly theophylline, remain widely used in some countries because of their low cost, although their benefit/ risk profiles are unfavorable compared with inhaled therapy. AAT augmentation therapy is useful in patients with AAT deficiency and progressive emphysema. Cardiovascular drugs should be used in COPD only if those patients have underlying cardiovascular condition supporting their indication. Ongoing research aims at identifying new therapeutic targets and agents in inflammation, destruction/repair mechanisms, immune regulation, microbiota homeostasis, mucus modulation, and lung regeneration.

REFERENCES

1. Global Initiative for Chronic Obstructive Lung Disease. Global strategy for the diagnosis, management and prevention of chronic obstructive lung disease. Available at: https://goldcopd.org.
2. Bagdonas E, Raudoniute J, Bruzauskaite I, et al. Novel aspects of pathogenesis and regeneration mechanisms in COPD. Int J Chron Obstruct Pulmon Dis 2015;10:995–1013.
3. Eapen MS, Myers S, Walters EH, et al. Airway inflammation in chronic obstructive pulmonary disease (COPD): a true paradox. Expert Rev Respir Med 2017;11:827–39.
4. Hussell T, Lui S, Jagger C, et al. The consequence of matrix dysfunction on lung immunity and the microbiome in COPD. Eur Respir Rev 2018;27. https://doi.org/10.1183/16000617.0032-2018.
5. Kesimer M, Ford AA, Ceppe A, et al. Airway mucin concentration as a marker of chronic bronchitis. N Engl J Med 2017;377:911–22.
6. Fischer BM, Voynow JA, Ghio AJ. COPD: balancing oxidants and antioxidants. Int J Chron Obstruct Pulmon Dis 2015;10:261–76.
7. Barnes PJ. Senescence in COPD and its comorbidities. Annu Rev Physiol 2017;79:517–39.

8. Caramori G, Ruggeri P, Di Stefano A, et al. Autoimmunity and COPD: clinical implications. Chest 2018;153:1424–31.

9. Barnes PJ, Celli BR. Systemic manifestations and comorbidities of COPD. Eur Respir J 2009;33:1165–85.

10. Rabe KF, Hurst JR, Suissa S. Cardiovascular disease and COPD: dangerous liaisons? Eur Respir Rev 2018;27. https://doi.org/10.1183/16000617.0057-2018.

11. Pelgrim CE, Peterson JD, Gosker HR, et al. Psychological co-morbidities in COPD: targeting systemic inflammation, a benefit for both? Eur J Pharmacol 2019;842:99–110.

12. Corlateanu A, Covantev S, Mathioudakis AG, et al. Prevalence and burden of comorbidities in chronic obstructive pulmonary disease. Respir Investig 2016;54:387–96.

13. Gimeno-Santos E, Frei A, Steurer-Stey C, et al. Determinants and outcomes of physical activity in patients with COPD: a systematic review. Thorax 2014. https://doi.org/10.1136/thoraxjnl-2013-204763.

14. Higham A, Quinn AM, Cançado JED, et al. The pathology of small airways disease in COPD: historical aspects and future directions. Respir Res 2019;20:49.

15. Cazzola M, Calderaro F, Califano C, et al. Oral bambuterol compared to inhaled salmeterol in patients with partially reversible chronic obstructive pulmonary disease. Eur J Clin Pharmacol 1999;54:829–33.

16. Shim CS, Williams MH. Bronchodilator response to oral aminophylline and terbutaline versus aerosol albuterol in patients with chronic obstructive pulmonary disease. Am J Med 1983;75:697–701.

17. Spina D, Page CP. Xanthines and phosphodiesterase inhibitors. Handb Exp Pharmacol 2017;237:63–91.

18. Pleasants RA. Clinical pharmacology of oral maintenance therapies for obstructive lung diseases. Respir Care 2018;63:671–89.

19. Cazzola M, Calzetta L, Barnes PJ, et al. Efficacy and safety profile of xanthines in COPD: a network meta-analysis. Eur Respir Rev 2018;27. https://doi.org/10.1183/16000617.0010-2018.

20. Barnes PJ. Theophylline. Am J Respir Crit Care Med 2013;188:901–6.

21. Cosio BG, Tsaprouni L, Ito K, et al. Theophylline restores histone deacetylase activity and steroid responses in COPD macrophages. J Exp Med 2004;200:689–95.

22. Barnes PJ, Adcock IM. Glucocorticoid resistance in inflammatory diseases. Lancet 2009;373:1905–17.

23. Ito K, Ito M, Elliott WM, et al. Decreased histone deacetylase activity in chronic obstructive pulmonary disease. N Engl J Med 2005;352:1967–76.

24. Devereux G, Cotton S, Fielding S, et al. Effect of theophylline as adjunct to inhaled corticosteroids on exacerbations in patients with COPD: a randomized clinical trial. JAMA 2018;320:1548–59.

25. Cosío BG, Shafiek H, Iglesias A, et al. Oral low-dose theophylline on top of inhaled fluticasone-salmeterol does not reduce exacerbations in patients with severe COPD: a pilot clinical trial. Chest 2016. https://doi.org/10.1016/j.chest.2016.04.011.

26. Compton CH, Gubb J, Nieman R, et al. Cilomilast, a selective phosphodiesterase-4 inhibitor for treatment of patients with chronic obstructive pulmonary disease: a randomised, dose-ranging study. Lancet 2001;358(9278):265–70, 358:265–70.

27. Lipworth BJ. Phosphodiesterase-4 inhibitors for asthma and chronic obstructive pulmonary disease. Lancet 2005;365:167–75.

28. Contreras S, Milara J, Morcillo E, et al. Selective inhibition of phosphodiesterases 4A, B, C and D isoforms in chronic respiratory diseases: current and future evidences. Curr Pharm Des 2017;23:2073–83.

29. Chong J, Leung B, Poole P. Phosphodiesterase 4 inhibitors for chronic obstructive pulmonary disease. Cochrane Database Syst Rev 2017;(9):CD002309.

30. Martinez FJ, Rabe KF, Sethi S, et al. Effect of roflumilast and inhaled corticosteroid/long-acting β2-agonist on chronic obstructive pulmonary disease exacerbations (RE(2)SPOND). a randomized clinical trial. Am J Respir Crit Care Med 2016;194:559–67.

31. Cazzola M, Calzetta L, Rogliani P, et al. Ensifentrine (RPL554): an investigational PDE3/4 inhibitor for the treatment of COPD. Expert Opin Investig Drugs 2019;28:827–33.

32. Albert RK, Connett J, Bailey WC, et al. Azithromycin for prevention of exacerbations of COPD. N Engl J Med 2011;365:689–98.

33. Uzun S, Djamin RS, Kluytmans JAJW, et al. Azithromycin maintenance treatment in patients with frequent exacerbations of chronic obstructive pulmonary disease (COLUMBUS): a randomised, double-blind, placebo-controlled trial. Lancet Respir Med 2014;2:361–8.

34. Seemungal TA, Wilkinson TM, Hurst JR, et al. Long-term erythromycin therapy is associated with decreased chronic obstructive pulmonary disease exacerbations. Am J Respir Crit Care Med 2008;178:1139–47.

35. Huckle AW, Fairclough LC, Todd I. Prophylactic antibiotic use in COPD and the potential anti-inflammatory activities of antibiotics. Respir Care 2018;63:609–19.

36. Cui Y, Luo L, Li C, et al. Long-term macrolide treatment for the prevention of acute exacerbations in COPD: a systematic review and meta-analysis. Int J Chron Obstruct Pulmon Dis 2018;13:3813–29.

37. Suzuki T, Yanai M, Yamaya M, et al. Erythromycin and common cold in COPD. Chest 2001;120:730–3.

38. Han MK, Tayob N, Murray S, et al. Predictors of chronic obstructive pulmonary disease

exacerbation reduction in response to daily azithromycin therapy. Am J Respir Crit Care Med 2014; 189:1503–8.

39. Sethi S, Jones PW, Theron MS, et al. Pulsed moxifloxacin for the prevention of exacerbations of chronic obstructive pulmonary disease: a randomized controlled trial. Respir Res 2010;11:10.

40. Decramer M, Janssens W. Mucoactive therapy in COPD. Eur Respir Rev 2010;19:134–40.

41. Cazzola M, Rogliani P, Calzetta L, et al. Impact of mucolytic agents on COPD exacerbations: a pairwise and network meta-analysis. COPD 2017;14: 552–63.

42. Manson SC, Brown RE, Cerulli A, et al. The cumulative burden of oral corticosteroid side effects and the economic implications of steroid use. Respir Med 2009;103:975–94.

43. Schols AM, Wesseling G, Kester AD, et al. Dose dependent increased mortality risk in COPD patients treated with oral glucocorticoids. Eur Respir J 2001;17(3):337–42.

44. Schols AM, Slangen J, Volovics L, et al. Weight loss is a reversible factor in the prognosis of chronic obstructive pulmonary disease. Am J Respir Crit Care Med 1998;157:1791–7.

45. Walters J, Walters E, Wood-Baker R. Oral corticosteroids for stable chronic obstructive pulmonary disease. Cochrane Database Syst Rev 2005;(3): CD005374.

46. Lee JH, Kim HJ, Kim YH. The effectiveness of antileukotriene agents in patients with COPD: a systemic review and meta-analysis. Lung 2015;193: 477–86.

47. Gottlieb SS, McCarter RJ, Vogel RA. Effect of betablockade on mortality among high-risk and low-risk patients after myocardial infarction. N Engl J Med 1998;339:489–97.

48. Dransfield MT, Voelker H, Bhatt SP, et al. Metoprolol for the prevention of acute exacerbations of COPD. N Engl J Med 2019;381:2304–14.

49. Criner GJ, Connett JE, Aaron SD, et al. Simvastatin for the prevention of exacerbations in moderate-to-severe COPD. N Engl J Med 2014;370:2201–10.

50. Parikh MA, Aaron CP, Hoffman EA, et al. Angiotensin-converting inhibitors and angiotensin II receptor blockers and longitudinal change in percent emphysema on computed tomography. The multiethnic study of atherosclerosis lung study. Ann Am Thorac Soc 2017;14:649–58.

51. Pavord ID. Biologics and chronic obstructive pulmonary disease. J Allergy Clin Immunol 2018;141: 1983–91.

52. Yousuf A, Brightling CE. Biologic drugs: a new target therapy in COPD? COPD 2018;15:99–107.

53. Woodruff PG, Agusti A, Roche N, et al. Current concepts in targeting chronic obstructive pulmonary disease pharmacotherapy: making progress towards personalised management. Lancet 2015; 385:1789–98.

54. Agusti A, Bel E, Thomas M, et al. Treatable traits: toward precision medicine of chronic airway diseases. Eur Respir J 2016;47:410–9.

55. Rennard SI, Flavin SK, Agarwal PK, et al. Long-term safety study of infliximab in moderate-to-severe chronic obstructive pulmonary disease. Respir Med 2013;107:424–32.

56. Dentener MA, Creutzberg EC, Pennings H-J, et al. Effect of infliximab on local and systemic inflammation in chronic obstructive pulmonary disease: a pilot study. Respiration 2008;76:275–82.

57. Pavord ID, Chanez P, Criner GJ, et al. Mepolizumab for eosinophilic chronic obstructive pulmonary disease. N Engl J Med 2017;377:1613–29.

58. Miravitlles M, Dirksen A, Ferrarotti I, et al. European Respiratory Society statement: diagnosis and treatment of pulmonary disease in α1-antitrypsin deficiency. Eur Respir J 2017;50. https://doi.org/10.1183/13993003.00610-2017.

59. Ahmadi Z, Bernelid E, Currow DC, et al. Prescription of opioids for breathlessness in end-stage COPD: a national population-based study. Int J Chron Obstruct Pulmon Dis 2016;11:2651–7.

60. Barnes H, McDonald J, Smallwood N, et al. Opioids for the palliation of refractory breathlessness in adults with advanced disease and terminal illness. Cochrane Database Syst Rev 2016;2016. https://doi.org/10.1002/14651858.CD011008.pub2.

Critical Analysis of the National Emphysema Treatment Trial Results for Lung-Volume-Reduction Surgery

Joseph J. Platz, MD*, Keith S. Naunheim, MD

KEYWORDS

- Emphysema • Lung-volume-reduction surgery • NETT • COPD • Thoracoscopy

KEY POINTS

- The National Emphysema Treatment Trial directly compared lung-volume-reduction surgery with maximal medical therapy for severe chronic obstructive pulmonary disease in a prospective randomized controlled fashion.
- The combination of a forced expiratory volume in 1 second (FEV_1) less than or equal to 20% of predicted with either homogeneous emphysema or diffusing capacity of the lungs for carbon monoxide (DLCO) less than or equal to 20% of predicted encompasses a group too high risk for surgery.
- In appropriately selected patients, surgery has a lower long-term mortality and improved exercise capacity compared with medical therapy, particularly in patients with upper-lobe emphysema and low pretreatment exercise capacity.
- Major pulmonary and cardiac morbidity occurs in 29.8% and 20.0% of patients, respectively with a 90-day mortality of 5.5%. Low FEV_1 and DLCO, non–upper-lobe emphysema, oral steroid use, and increased age are correlated to these complications.

INTRODUCTION

Chronic obstructive pulmonary disease (COPD) is one of the leading causes of mortality in the United States. In 2015 there were 15.5 million adults diagnosed with the lower respiratory disease with 335,000 Medicare hospitalizations and 150,350 associated deaths.[1] Medical treatment consists of a combination of inhaled corticosteroids, bronchodilators, oxygen, and pulmonary rehabilitation. Despite treatment, mortality remains minimally changed over the past 30 years at approximately 40 deaths per 100,000 US population.[2] As early as 1950, surgical lung resection of diseased lung was proposed as potentially beneficial COPD treatment. However, prohibitively high morbidity and mortality caused the procedure to fall out of favor.[3] Lung-volume-reduction surgery (LVRS) was reborn in 2003 when Joel Cooper and colleagues[4] demonstrated the ability to significantly improve outcomes of targeted lung resection by taking advantage of 40 years worth of advances in technology, technique, anesthesia, critical care, and rehabilitation.

The overall goal of LVRS is removal of emphysematous lung in order to enhance overall pulmonary function. Multiple mechanisms have been credited with this beneficial enhancement, including improvements in pulmonary elastic recoil, diaphragmatic function, left ventricular filling, endothelial health, as well as decreased functional residual

Division of Cardiothoracic Surgery, Saint Louis University School of Medicine, 1008 South Spring Avenue, Saint Louis, MO 63110, USA
* Corresponding author.
E-mail address: Joe.platz@health.slu.edu

Thorac Surg Clin 31 (2021) 107–118
https://doi.org/10.1016/j.thorsurg.2021.01.004

thoracic.theclinics.com

capacity and intrathoracic pressure.[5–8] Single-institution studies initially published demonstrated significant variation in operative mortality (2.5%–19%) with 1-year mortality as high as 23%.[9,10] Uncertainty around the operative morbidity, mortality, magnitude of benefit, duration of improvement, and prognostic predictors of LVRS led to the creation of the National Emphysema Treatment Trial (NETT). This federally funded, multicenter study was created to directly compare LVRS with maximal medical therapy for severe emphysema in a randomized controlled fashion.[11] Much of our current treatment of COPD is still based on this trial.

NATIONAL EMPHYSEMA TREATMENT TRIAL

The NETT was initiated in 1998 in order to clarify the benefit of LVRS. Previously published studies on the efficacy of LVRS were relatively small and included patient cohorts with differing clinical characteristics operated on using various surgical techniques. Almost all studies lacked long-term follow-up and did not comprehensively assess benefit, risk, or cost. NETT sought to reduce the variability in patient characteristics, surgical technique, patient care, and follow-up with the creation of a multiinstitution randomized study. Given the lack of clarity surrounding both the risk and the benefit of surgical intervention, both were evaluated as the study's primary outcome measures. Survival was chosen as a primary outcome, given its ease and accuracy of measurement as well as its clinical significance in a population with emphysema and a resultant high baseline mortality. The other primary outcome measurement was exercise capacity as determined by cycle ergometry. This was chosen over other modalities due to its reproducibility, standardization, and administration. In addition, exercise capacity was favored over pulmonary function testing (PFT), as the latter had not demonstrated a consistent relationship with functional status. A 10-W change in exercise performance and an 8-point change in St. George Respiratory Questionnaire were deemed meaningful clinical changes in exercise capacity. The trial also looked at several secondary outcomes including quality of life (Medical Outcomes Study 36-Item Short Form and Quality of Well-Being Scale), cost, complications, PFTs, radiologic volumetric analysis, 6-minute walk distance, cardiovascular measures, and psychomotor function.

The study was designed as a randomized controlled non-crossover comparison of maximal medical therapy with medical therapy plus LVRS in patients with severe. Patients were randomized in a 1:1 fashion between treatment groups and then within the surgery group were randomized further between median sternotomy and video-assisted thoracoscopic surgery (VATS) in those institutions capable of performing both. Seventeen centers participated in the trial in total, with 8 performing sternotomies only, 3 performing VATS only, and 6 randomizing between the two. Regardless of the approach, the goal was to resect 20% to 35% of bilateral lungs, targeting the most diseased portions.[12] Patients were required to have severe COPD with a forced expiratory volume in 1 second (FEV_1) less than or equal to 45%, a total lung capacity greater than or equal to 100%, a residual volume (RV) greater than or equal to 150%, and $Paco_2$ less than or equal to 60 mm Hg. They were additionally expected to have quit smoking for more than 4 months and to have attended pulmonary rehabilitation for at least 6 to 10 weeks before intervention. Exclusion criteria included prior major lung surgery and/or infection, significant cardiac disease, severe obesity, recent malignancy, 6-minute walk less than 140 m after rehabilitation, or another significant comorbidity.[13]

Before treatment, patient demographics, pulmonary function, imaging, functional status, exercise capacity, and quality of life were measured. Full assessment was repeated at 6 months, 12 months, and then yearly.[11] As a safety measure, at the onset of the study, the monitoring board was providing stopping guidelines to be used to identify those that were clearly benefited and those that were clearly harmed by LVRS. An 8% 30-day mortality was used as the cutoff of unacceptable risk. Initially those predicted to benefit most from surgical intervention were those younger than 70 years with FEV_1 between 15% and 35% of predicted, $Paco_2$ less than 50 mm Hg, RV greater than 200% of predicted, and with a heterogeneous pattern of emphysema with minimal perfusion. These variables were monitored by the board as well as diffusing capacity of the lungs for carbon monoxide (DLCO), work capacity, quality of life, race, and sex. In addition to the regular assessments discussed earlier, these variables were reviewed every 3 months for signs of clear patient benefit or risk. In April of 2001 low FEV_1, homogeneous emphysema, a high perfusion ratio, and low DLCO demonstrated an increased risk of mortality. Additional analyses were performed to define if these parameters met the unacceptable risk criteria. They found that the combination of an FEV_1 less than or equal to 20% of predicted with either homogeneous emphysema or DLCO less than or equal to 20% of predicted led to an 18% 30-day surgical mortality compared with zero deaths in the medical arm of the study. These groups were labeled as "high risk" and subsequently excluded from the trial.[13]

NETT continued to accrue until 2002, and by 2003 the first complete analysis was performed. In total 1218 patient were randomized out of 3777 evaluated, with 608 in the surgery arm and 610 in the medical arm. One hundred forty of these patients were in the preexclusion high-risk group with 42 and 30 in the surgical and medical arms, respectively. Baseline characteristics were similar between both treatment arms except that there was a higher proportion of men in the medical-therapy arm.[11] Initial, analysis looked at the primary outcomes over the 4-year trial period and with a mean patient follow-up of 2.4 years. Over the following years, subsequent analyses looked at NETT's secondary outcomes and were eventually followed by an updated publication of the primary outcomes. This latter long-term analysis published in 2006 had a median patient follow-up of 4.3 years with 40% more 2-year-postrandomization data than the initial report.[14]

PRIMARY OUTCOMES
Mortality

On initial analysis, 90-day mortality was revealed to be 7.9% (95% confidence interval, 5.9–10.3) in the surgery group, significantly higher than the 1.3% (95% confidence interval, 0.6–2.6) of the medical group ($P<.001$). This was however considered expected, given the immediate trauma of surgery and overall mortality was not significantly different between groups with a total morality of 0.11 deaths per person-year in both treatment arms. When the previously discussed high-risk group was removed from the analysis, 90-day mortality was 5.2% in the surgical arm compared with 1.5% in the medical arm, whereas overall mortality was 0.09 and 0.10 deaths per person-year, respectively ($P = .31$) (**Table 1**).[11] Interestingly, despite increased early mortality in the LVRS arm, long-term analysis in 2006 demonstrated that total mortality was 0.11 deaths per person-year in the surgery group versus 0.13 in the medical group, a statistically significant difference ($P = .02$). This benefit of surgery remained with removal of the high-risk group from analysis with 0.10 and 0.12 deaths per person-year, respectively. In subgroup analysis, mortality was reviewed in relation to the distribution of emphysema as well as exercise capacity. The 2003 initial analysis found that surgery most benefited patients with upper-lobe–predominant emphysema and low pretreatment exercise capacity. In this group, 90-day mortality was no different between the LVRS and medical arms (2.9% vs 3.3%,

$P = 1.0$), and total mortality was significantly better after undergoing surgery (0.07 vs 0.15 death per person-year, $P = .005$). This benefit continued in the long-term follow-up (**Fig. 1**). In patients with non–upper-lobe emphysema, 90-day mortality was significantly higher in the surgery group regardless of exercise capacity, and total mortality was significantly higher for those with a high exercise capacity.[15]

Exercise Capacity

Exercise capacity was measured by ergometer and a change of 10 W after treatment was considered clinically significant. At 6, 12, and 24 months of follow-up the surgery group improved in exercise capacity by more than 10 W in 28%, 22%, and 15% of patients, respectively. This is compared with 4%, 5%, and 3% in the medicine group. Although the LVRS group demonstrated an initial improvement in function after the immediate postoperative period, outcome measures showed a progressive decline in capacity over time, as the medical therapy group. Long-term analysis evidenced that trend with the surgery group displaying an over-10 W improvement in 23%, 15%, and 9% compared with 5%, 3%, and 1% in medicine group at 1, 2, and 3 years. In both time frames, the values were statistically significant between treatment arms (**Table 2**). In addition, although not a primary outcome measurement, analyses analyzed St. George's Respiratory Questionnaire (SGRQ) results in addition to ergometry to assess exercise capacity. Clinically significant improvement was determined to be an over-8-unit decrease on the questionnaire. In the LVRS group, said improvement was noted in 40%, 32%, 20%, 10%, and 13% at 1, 2, 3, 4, and 5 years after randomization compared with 9%, 8%, 8%, 4%, and 7% in the medical group at similar intervals; these differences were significant through the first 4 years ($P<.001$, years 1–3; $P = .005$, year 4). In subgroup analysis by emphysema distribution and exercise capacity, those with upper-lobe disease and low pretreatment exercise capacity had the highest likelihood of greater than 10 W capacity improvement and the most benefit at 24 months compared with the medical group (30% vs 0%, $P<.001$). Those with upper-lobe disease and high pretreatment capacity also had statistically significant improvement compared with the medical group but less so (15% vs 3% >10 W change, $P = .001$). Improvement of exercise capacity was similar between treatment arms in those with non–upper-lobe disease (**Fig. 2**). Long-term analysis continued to support these findings and additionally

Table 1
Ninety-day and total mortality among all patients and non–high-risk subgroups at 3 years

	90-Day Mortality			Total Mortality					
	Surgery Group	Medical-Therapy Group		Surgery Group		Medical-Therapy Group			
Patients	No. of Deaths/Total no. (% [95% CI])	No. of Deaths/Total no. (% [95% CI])	P Value	No. of Deaths/ Total no.	No. Of Deaths/ Person-Year	No. of Deaths/ Total no.	No. of Deaths/ Person-Year	Risk Ratio	P Value
All patients	48/608 (7.9 [5.9–10.3])	8/610 (1.3 [0.6–2.6])	<.001	157/608	0.11	160/610	0.11	1.01	0.90
High-risk[†]	20/70 (28.6 [18.4–40.6])	0/70 (0 [0–5.1])	<.001	42/70	0.33	30/70	0.18	1.82	0.06
Other[‡]	28/538 (5.2(3.5–7.4])	8/540 (1.5 [0.6–2.9])	.001	115/538	0.09	130/540	0.10	0.89	0.31
Subgroups[‡]									
Patients with predominantly upper-lobe emphysema									
Low exercise capacity	4/139 (2.9 [0.8–7.2])	5/151 (3.3 [1.1–7.6])	1.00	26/139	0.07	51/151	0.15	0.47	0.005
High exercise capacity	6/206 (2.9 [1.1–6.2])	2/213 (0.9 [0.1–3.4])	.17	34/206	0.07	39/213	0.07	0.98	0.70
Patients with predominantly non-upper-lobe emphysema									
Low exercise capacity	7/84 (8.3 [3.4–16.4])	0/65 (0 [0–5.5])	.02	28/84	0.15	26/65	0.18	0.81	0.49
High exercise capacity	11/109 (10.1 [5.1–17.3])	1/111 (0.9 [0.02–4.9])	.003	27/109	0.10	14/111	0.05	2.06	0.02

Mean patient follow-up of 29.2 months.

[†] High-risk patients were defined as those with a forced expiratory volume in one second (FEV1) that was 20 percent or less of the predicted value and either homogeneous emphysema on computed tomography or a carbon monoxide diffusing capacity that was 20 percent or less of the predicted value.

[‡] High-risk patients were excluded from the subgroup analyses. For total mortality, P for interaction=0.004; this P value was derived from binary logistic-regression models with terms for treatment, subgroup, and the interaction between the two, with the use of an exact-score test with three degrees of freedom. Other factors that were considered as potential variables for the definition of subgroups included the base-line FEV1, carbon monoxide diffusing capacity, partial pressure of arterial carbon dioxide, residual volume, ratio of residual volume to total lung capacity, ratio of expired ventilation in one minute to carbon dioxide excretion in one minute, distribution of emphysema (heterogeneous vs. homogeneous), perfusion ratio, score for health-related quality of life, and Quality of Well-Being score; age; race or ethnic group; and sex.

From National Emphysema Treatment Trial Research Group. A randomized trial comparing lung-volume-reduction surgery with medical therapy for severe emphysema. N Engl J Med 2003;348:2059–2073; with permission.

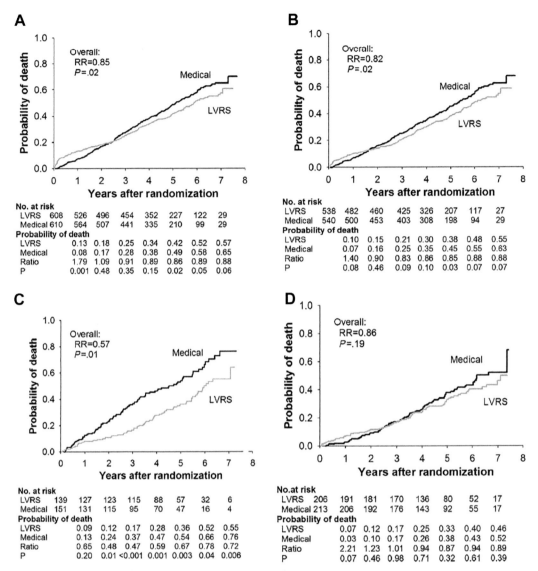

Fig. 1. Kaplan-Meier curves representing the cumulative probability of death after randomization of LVRS and medical treatment groups. (*A*) All patients. (*B*) Non–high-risk patients. (*C*) Upper-lobe–-predominant, low exercise capacity. (*D*) Upper-lobe–predominant, high exercise capacity. (*From* Naunheim KS, Wood DE, Mohsenifar Z, et al. Long-term follow-up of patients receiving lung-volume-reduction surgery versus medical therapy for severe emphysema by the national emphysema treatment trial research group. Ann Thorac Surg 2006;82:431-443; with permission.)

demonstrated significant improvements in SGRQ score with surgery compared with medical treatment. Statistical significance was maintained through 5 years in patients with upper-lobe, low exercise capacity, 4 years in patients with upper-lobe high exercise capacity, and 3 years in patients with non–upper-lobe low exercise capacity. Patients with non–upper-lobe high exercise capacity were similarly unlikely to have improvement in SGRQ regardless of treatment.[11,15]

SECONDARY OUTCOMES
Six-Minute Walk Distance Reproducibility

Exercise capacity as measured by ergometry was used as a primary respiratory outcome measure in NETT but 6-minute walk distance was also analyzed as a secondary outcome. This test is commonly used in practice to measure functional and exercise capacity. Although it has been somewhat standardized, there is lack of consensus on the importance of course length, shape, or the

Table 2
Improvement in exercise capacity and health-related quality of life as measured by the St. George's Respiratory Questionnaire in all patients and non–high-risk subgroups at 24 months postrandomization

Patients	Improvement in Exercise Capacity				Improvement in Health-Related Quality of Life			
	Surgery Group no./Total no. (%)	Medical-Therapy Group no./Total no. (%)	Odds Ratio	P Value	Surgery Group no./Total no. (%)	Medical-Therapy Group no./Total no. (%)	Odds Ratio	P Value
All patients	54/371 (15)	10/378 (3)	6.27	<.001	121/371 (33)	34/378 (9)	4.90	<.001
High-risk[†]	4/58 (7)	1/48 (2)	3.48	.37	6/58 (10)	0/48	—	.03
Other	50/313 (16)	9/330 (3)	6.78	<.001	115/313 (37)	34/330 (10)	5.06	<.001
Subgroups[‡]								
Predominantly upper-lobe emphysema								
Low exercise capacity	25/84 (30)	0/92	—	<.001	40/84 (48)	9/92 (10)	8.38	<.001
High exercise capacity	17/115 (15)	4/138 (3)	5.81	.001	47/115 (41)	15/138 (11)	5.67	<.001
Predominantly non-upper-lobe emphysema								
Low exercise capacity	6/49 (12)	3/41 (7)	1.77	.50	18/49 (37)	3/41 (7)	7.35	.001
High exercise capacity	2/65 (3)	2/59 (3)	0.90	1.00	10/65 (15)	7/59 (12)	1.35	.61

Improvement in exercise capacity defined as an increase on ergometry of greater than 10 W or a decrease on the questionnaire of greater than 8 units from pretreatment baselines.
[†] High-risk patients were defined as those with a forced expiratory volume in one second (FEV1) that was 20 percent or less of the predicted value and either homogeneous emphysema on computed tomography or a carbon monoxide diffusing capacity that was 20 percent or less of the predicted value.
[‡] High-risk patients were excluded from the subgroup analyses. For improvement in exercise capacity, P for interaction=0.005; for improvement in health-related quality of life, P for interaction=0.03. These P values were derived from binary logistic-regression models with terms for treatment, subgroup, and the interaction between the two, with the use of an exact-score test with three degrees of freedom. Other factors that were considered as potential variables for the definition of subgroups included the base-line FEV1, carbon monoxide diffusing capacity, partial pressure of arterial carbon dioxide, residual volume, ratio of residual volume to total lung capacity, ratio of expired ventilation in one minute to carbon dioxide excretion in one minute, distribution of emphysema (heterogeneous vs. homogeneous), perfusion ratio, score for healthrelated quality of life, and Quality of Well-Being score; age; race or ethnic group; and sex.
From National Emphysema Treatment Trial Research Group. A randomized trial comparing lung-volume-reduction surgery with medical therapy for severe emphysema. N Engl J Med 2003;348:2059–2073; with permission.

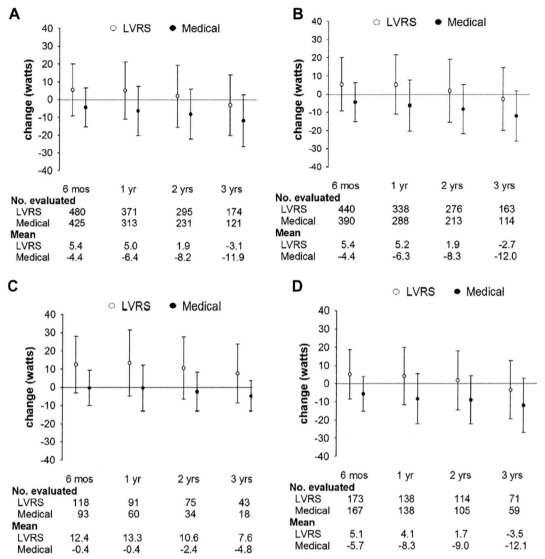

Fig. 2. Mean change in exercise capacity from pretreatment baseline as measured at 6 months, 1 year, 2 years, and 3 years between LVRS and medical treatment groups. Numbers reflect number of patients evaluated and mean change. Error bars represent the standard deviation of change. (*A*) All patients. (*B*) Non–high-risk patients. (*C*) Upper-lobe–predominant, low exercise capacity. (*D*) Upper-lobe–predominant, high exercise capacity. (*From* Naunheim KS, Wood DE, Mohsenifar Z, et al. Long-term follow-up of patients receiving lung-volume-reduction surgery versus medical therapy for severe emphysema by the national emphysema treatment trial research group. Ann Thorac Surg 2006;82:431-443; with permission.)

role of practice/second walk. Four hundred seventy of the NETT participants at 17 institutions were asked to undergo a 6-minute walk test as well as a second test the following day. The test was reproducible on subsequent days but with a clear learning effect. Walked distance was greater on the second day by an average of 66.1 feet (*P*<.0001) or 7%. Seventy percent of people improved the on second day with the greatest improvements generally accomplished by those with greater first-day distances. Track length did not

seem to influence walking distance; however, participants who used a continuous looped track performed better than those on a straight track (1156 feet vs 1266 feet, *P* = .003).[16]

Air Leak

Unlike with traditional anatomic lung resection, air leak after LVRS can be difficult to control due to the degree of lung emphysema and the long parenchymal staple lines. As such, LVRS was often performed with buttressed or reinforced staple lines even though true effectiveness in reducing air leak was unclear. Five hundred fifty-two of the NETT LVRS patients had detailed 30-day postoperative air leak data analyzed with attention paid to operative technique, leak prevalence and duration, and medical consequences. Of the patients evaluated, 90% experienced an air leak at some time during their 30-day postoperative course with a slightly increased risk in those with low DLCO and a decreased risk with a lower lobe staple line. The mean duration of air leak was 7 days, but 66 of the 493 affected patients had an air leak for at least 30 days. Leaks lasted significantly longer in Caucasians, those with low DLCO or FEV_1, those with pleural adhesions, those using inhaled steroids, or those who primarily underwent upper-lobe resection. The use of staple line buttress or the type of buttress did not seem to influence the presence or duration of an air leak. Thirty-day mortality was similar between those that did and did not experience an air leak (4% vs 0%, $P = .11$), but 4.4% of patients with a leak required reoperation and the postoperative complication rate was significantly higher in those who experienced an air leak after propensity matching (57% vs 30%, $P = .004$). Pneumonia and intensive care unit (ICU) readmission were the most severe complications in this group. Lastly, the length of stay in 30-day survivors was longer for those who experienced an air leak (11.8 ± 6.5 days vs 7.6 ± 4.4 days, $P = .0005$).[17]

Pulmonary Rehabilitation

As part of the inclusion criteria for NETT, all patients were required to undergo pretreatment pulmonary rehabilitation. This allowed for patient optimization but also for evaluation of the effectiveness of rehabilitation and analysis of its benefit. Of the 1218 studied patients, 777 (64%) had received pulmonary rehabilitation before the trial and 58% required supplemental oxygen to maintain saturation over 90%. Pulmonary rehabilitation consistently led to significant improvements in exercise capacity, dyspnea, and quality of life measures with more benefit noted in those that had not undergone prior rehabilitation. Approximately half of patients met what was considered clinically important improvements with pulmonary rehabilitation (cycle workload of 5 W, SGRQ score of 4 units, UCSD Shortness of Breath Questionnaire score of 5 units). Overall, 20% of non–high-risk patients changed exercise capacity subgroup after pulmonary rehabilitation, with 13.5% changing from low- to high-capacity subgroups. The effect was even higher for patients without prior rehabilitation experience, with 16.5% changing from

the low exercise capacity subgroup to the high exercise capacity subgroup. Functional improvements with pulmonary rehabilitation did not significantly correlate with primary NETT outcome measurements nor objective functional lung improvements; however, it was thought that the pulmonary rehabilitation experience optimized preoperative physical and emotional function as well as helped to exclude those too unhealthy for randomization.[18]

Surgical Approach

After pulmonary rehabilitation, patients were randomized in a 1:1 fashion either into the medical treatment group or into the LVRS group. Within the surgical group, 8 clinical centers performed surgery only by median sternotomy, 3 only by VATS, and at the remaining 6 centers, patients were again randomized 1:1 to either sternotomy or VATS. In total, of the 608 surgically randomized patients, 511 remained after exclusions and removal of the high-risk group, of which 359 patients underwent resection by median sternotomy and 152 by VATS. Patient characteristics were similar between groups other than slightly more heterogeneous emphysema in the sternotomy group (61% vs 51%, $P = .04$). Surgeons estimated larger resections with sternotomy but that was not supported by specimen weight nor was there a difference when analysis was limited to the randomization centers. Mortality was no different between techniques, with 90-day mortality of 5.9% for sternotomy and 4.6% for VATS ($P = .67$) and total mortality of 0.08 and 0.10 deaths per person-year, respectively ($P = .42$). When looking at all centers, VATS cases were 20% longer ($P<.001$), had a higher likelihood of intraoperative hypoxemia ($P = .004$), had a higher rate of postoperative air leak ($P = .05$), and required fewer ICU days ($P<.001$). However, none of these factors were statistically significant when comparison was restricted to the 6 centers that randomized surgical technique. Median length of stay was 1 day longer for sternotomy ($P = .01$), and 30-day independent living was higher in the VATS group. This latter measurement, however, became nonsignificant by 4 months postoperatively. There were no differences in exercise capacity or lung function by approach. Interestingly, both initial hospital costs and 6-month costs were significantly lower for the VATS groups by almost 20% (hospital: $38557 vs $30350, $P = .03$; 6 month: $61481 vs $51053, $P = .005$).[19]

Cost

Cost is always a difficult measure to analyze in terms of treatment, particularly over the course of time. The NETT group conducted a cost-effectiveness analysis to determine the cost per quality-adjusted life-year gained in the non–high-risk group. They estimated the "cost" of medical goods and services (Medicare charges), transportation, time spent by family and friends caring for the patient, and time spent by the patient undergoing treatment. These costs were correlated to quality-adjusted life-years through use of the Quality of Well-Being questionnaire. After several exclusions, 531 surgical and 535 medical patients were analyzed with near identical pretreatment Quality of Well-Being scores of 0.58 and 0.57, respectively. Expectedly, over the first-year postrandomization, the surgery group had significantly more hospital days (24.9 vs 4.9), ambulatory care days (10.3 vs 8.6), and nursing home admissions (0.1 vs 0.0) than the medical group ($P \leq .005$). Over the next year however, hospital days were lower in the LVRS group (3.2 vs 6.1, $P = .005$) as were emergency-room visits (0.5 vs 0.7, $P = .04$). No differences in health care utilization were noted in the final year of follow-up. Both direct medical costs and total health care–related costs were significantly higher in the surgery group over the first year of follow-up, with the latter being $71,515 versus $23,371 in the medical group ($P<.001$). Again, this relationship inverts between 13 and 24 months postrandomization, with the medical group incurring nearly twice the total costs of the surgical group in the second year. There was no statistical difference in costs between 25 and 36 months postrandomization. Finally, despite initially higher costs and medical utilization, quality-adjusted life-years gained were significantly higher in the surgical group (1.46 vs 1.27, $P<.001$). This was further evaluated through subgroup (disease location and exercise capacity) analysis. The subgroup with non–upper-lobe emphysema and high pretreatment exercise capacity had significantly higher mortality, costs, and reduced quality-adjusted survival after LVRS. In the other 3 subgroups, however, although total costs were significantly higher in the surgical arms ($P<.001$), quality-adjusted life-years gained were consistently higher after LVRS. As in the other analyses, the subgroup with upper-lobe disease and low exercise capacity faired best with the least cost difference compared with the medical group ($98,952 vs $62,560) as well as the biggest improvement in quality-adjusted survival in years (1.54 vs 1.04, $P<.001$) (**Table 3**).[20]

Operative Morbidity and Mortality Prediction

Even with appropriate patient selection, the risk and complication rate of LVRS is high. The NETT group analyzed 511 non–high-risk patients from the surgery arm of the trial in an attempt to identify predictors of operative morbidity and mortality. Intraoperative complications were rare, with hypoxia being the most common at 2.2%. Thirty-day morbidity on the other hand was high at almost 60%, composed mostly of arrhythmia and respiratory failure, the latter including need for reintubation, prolonged ventilation, ICU readmission, and tracheostomy. Overall, major pulmonary and cardiac morbidity occurred in 29.8% and 20.0% of patients respectively with a 90-day mortality of 5.5%. These data were correlated with patient characteristics followed by logistic regression with backward selection analysis. Ninety-day mortality was only found to be significantly associated with non–upper-lobe emphysematous disease as read by a radiologist ($P = .009$). Thirty-day postoperative pulmonary morbidity was significantly related to age ($P = .02$), FEV_1 percent predicted ($P = .05$), and DLCO percent predicted ($P = .01$). Cardiac morbidity over the same time course was significantly associated with steroid use ($P = .04$), non–upper-lobe disease by software analysis ($P<.001$), and age ($P = .004$). These predictors of morbidity and mortality correlate well with other subgroups analyses of LVRS risk and benefit.[21]

The National Emphysema Treatment Trial Success

The NETT was the first large prospective randomized investigation into the effectiveness and benefit of LVRS. Its initial and subsequent analyses added significant understanding and guidance to our treatment of severe emphysematous lung disease. NETT defined the ideal LVRS-patient population and, as such, demonstrated how preoperative lung function, exercise capacity, and emphysema distribution affect patient outcomes. Further, the large multiinstitutional nature of the trial allowed analyses of several important secondary outcomes that would not have been possible otherwise; some of these have broad implications outside of LVRS. Lastly, although initial studies showed a high mortality with LVRS, after refined patient selection, surgery led not only to significantly greater survival compared with nonoperative management but also to both improvements in functional status and quality of life. The NETT, with its rigorous study design and data collection, serves as the backbone for current and future investigation into the interventional treatment of advanced emphysema.

The National Emphysema Treatment Trial Failure

Despite these demonstrated benefits however, the biggest criticism of NETT was its inability to translate statistical data into clinical practice and

Table 3
Total health care–related costs, quality-adjusted life-years gained, and estimated cost-effectiveness of LVRS and medical treatment in all patients and non–high-risk subgroups at 3 years

Variable	Surgery Group		Medical-Therapy Group		P Value	Incremental Cost-Effectiveness Ratio for Surgery ($)
	No. of Patients	Mean (95% CI)	No. of Patients	Mean (95% CI)		
All patients	531		535			
Total costs ($)		98,952 (91,694–106,210)		62,560 (56,572–68,547)	<0.001	190,000
Quality-adjusted life-years gained		1.46 (1.46–1.47)		1.27 (1.27–1.28)	<0.001	
Patients with predominantly upper-lobe emphysema and low exercise capacity	137		148			98,000
Total costs ($)		110,815 (93,404–128,226)		61,804 (50,248–73,359)	<0.001	
Quality-adjusted life-years gained		1.54 (1.53–1.55)		1.04 (1.03–1.05)	<0.001	
Patients with predominantly upper-lobe emphysema and high exercise capacity	204		212			240,000
Total costs ($)		84,331 (73,699–94,962)		55,858 (47,161–64,555)	<0.001	
Quality-adjusted life-years gained		1.54 (1.54–1.55)		1.42 (1.42–1.43)	<0.001	
Patients with non–upper-lobe emphysema and low exercise capacity	82		65			330,000
Total costs ($)		111,986 (93,944–130,027)		65,655 (52,075–79,236)	<0.001	
Quality-adjusted life-years gained		1.25 (1.23–1.26)		1.10 (1.09–1.12)	<0.001	

From National Emphysema Treatment Trial Research Group. Cost effectiveness of lung-volume-reduction surgery for patients with severe emphysema. N Engl J Med 2003;348(21):2092-2102; with permission.

convince both surgeons and referring physicians of the possible role of LVRS. The number of people undergoing LVRS continues to be low and is likely decreasing. Reasons for this trend are not entirely clear but have been attributed to several factors. Firstly, the initial publications out of the trial noted a high overall mortality. NETT included a population of patients who were known to be high risk even before the study and therefore whose outcomes tainted the trial's results somewhat, but more importantly, left a negative connotation of LVRS among the nonsurgical community. Even though further analyses emphasized improved survival with appropriate patient selection, the high-risk nature of LVRS was hard for many to overlook. Given the pretrial suspicion, this high-risk population likely should have never been part of the study. Secondly, although NETT publications throughout the years have helped to define the ideal LVRS patient, what constitutes an appropriate surgical candidate is not clear to the medical community as a whole.[14] This is furthered by the fact that current LVRS is not always adherent to NETT inclusion criteria and as such demonstrates variable risk and benefit.[22] Lastly, restricting LVRS to certain approved centers (NETT, lung transplant, or Joint Commission on Accreditation of Healthcare Organizations–accredited centers), with the requirement for availability-limited pulmonary rehabilitation, makes surgical referral time-consuming, overly complicated, and detrimental to patient access.

CLINICS CARE POINTS

- Lung volume reduction surgery reduces mortality and improves exercise capacity in appropriately selected emphysematous patients compared to medical therapy alone.
- LVRS is most beneficial to those with heterogeneous localized emphysema and a decreased pre-operative exercise capacity.
- Surgery is not recommended for those with either FEV1 or DLCO less than or equal to 20% of predicted.

DISCLOSURE

The authors have no commercial, financial, or other conflicts of interest to disclose.

REFERENCES

1. Croft JB, Wheaton AG, Liu Y, et al. Urban-rural county and state differences in chronic obstructive pulmonary disease - United States. 2015. MMWR Morb Mortal Wkly Rep 2018;67(7):205–11.

2. Prevention Center for Disease Control and National. COPD death rates in the United States. Vital Statistics System 2018. Available at: https://www.cdc.gov/copd/data.html. Accessed July 6, 2020.

3. Deslauriers J. History of surgery for emphysema. Semin Thorac Cardiovasc Surg 1996;8:43–51.

4. Cooper JD, Trulock EP, Triantafillou AN, et al. Bilateral pneumectomy (volume reduction) for chronic obstructive pulmonary disease. J Thorac Cardiovasc Surg 1995;109(1):106–19.

5. Sciurba FC, Rogers RM, Keenan RJ, et al. Improvement in pulmonary function and elastic recoil after lung-reduction surgery for diffuse emphysema. N Engl J Med 1996;334:1095.

6. Lando Y, Boiselle PM, Shade D, et al. Effect of lung volume reduction surgery on diaphragm length in severe chronic obstructive pulmonary disease. Am J Respir Crit Care Med 1999;159:796.

7. Jörgensen K, Houltz E, Westfelt U, et al. Effects of lung volume reduction surgery on left ventricular diastolic filling and dimensions in patients with severe emphysema. Chest 2003;124:1863.

8. Clarenbach CF, Sievi NA, Brock M, et al. Lung volume reduction surgery and improvement of endothelial function and blood pressure in patients with Chronic Obstructive Pulmonary Disease. A randomized controlled trial. Am J Respir Crit Care Med 2015;192:307.

9. Health Care Financing Administration. Report to congress: lung volume reduction surgery and Medicare coverage policy-implications of recently published evidence. Washington, DC: Department of Health and Human Services; 1998.

10. DeCamp MM, McKenna RJ, Deschamps CC, et al. Lung volume reduction surgery: technique, operative mortality, and morbidity. Proc Am Thorac Soc 2008;5:442–6.

11. National Emphysema Treatment Trial Research Group. A randomized trial comparing lung-volume-reduction surgery with medical therapy for severe emphysema. N Engl J Med 2003;348:2059–73.

12. National Emphysema Treatment Trial Research Group. Rationale and design of the national emphysema treatment trial (NETT): a prospective randomized trial of lung volume reduction surgery. J Thorac Cardiovasc Surg 1999;118:518–28.

13. National Emphysema Treatment Trial Research Group. Patients at high risk of death after lung-volume-reduction surgery. N Engl J Med 2001;345(15):1075–83.

14. Criner GJ, Cordova F, Sternberg AL, et al. The national emphysema treatment trial (NETT) - Part II: lessons learned about lung volume reduction surgery. Am J Respir Crit Care Med 2011;184:881–93.

15. Naunheim KS, Wood DE, Mohsenifar Z, et al. Long-term follow-up of patients receiving lung-volume-reduction surgery versus medical therapy for severe emphysema by the national emphysema treatment trial research group. Ann Thorac Surg 2006;82: 431–43.

16. Sciurba F, Criner GJ, Lee SM, et al. Six-minute walk distance in chronic obstructive pulmonary disease: reproducibility and effect of walking course layout and layout. Am J Respir Crit Care Med 2003;167: 1522–7.

17. DeCamp MM, Blackstone EH, Naunheim KS, et al. Patient and surgical factors influencing air leak after lung volume reduction surgery: lessons learned from the national emphysema treatment trial. Ann Thorac Surg 2006;82:197–207.

18. Ries AL, Make BJ, Lee SM, et al. The effects of pulmonary rehabilitation in the national emphysema treatment trial. Chest 2005;128(6):3799–809.

19. National Emphysema Treatment Trial Research Group. Safety and efficacy of median sternotomy versus video-assisted thoracic surgery for lung volume reduction surgery. J Thorac Cardiovasc Surg 2004;127:1350–60.

20. National Emphysema Treatment Trial Research Group. Cost effectiveness of lung-volume-reduction surgery for patients with severe emphysema. N Engl J Med 2003;348(21):2092–102.

21. Naunheim KS, Wood DE, Krasna MJ, et al. Predictors of operative mortality and cardiopulmonary morbidity in the national emphysema treatment trial. J Thorac Cardiovasc Surg 2006;131(1):43–53.

22. Decker MR, Leverson GE, Jaoude WA, et al. Lung volume reduction surgery since the national emphysema treatment trial: study of society of thoracic surgeons database. J Thorac Cardiovasc Surg 2014;148(6):2651–8.

Analysis of Recent Literature on Lung Volume Reduction Surgery

Daniel P. McCarthy, MD, MBA, MEM[a], Lauren J. Taylor, MD[b],
Malcolm M. DeCamp, MD[c],*

KEYWORDS

- Emphysema • Lung volume reduction surgery • COPD

KEY POINTS

- LVRS may enact clinical benefit through improvements in chest wall asynchrony, increased maximum inspiratory pressure, and reduction in inflammatory mediators.
- Recent data demonstrate that LVRS may be performed safely with 6-month mortality of 0% to 1.5% and durable functional improvements.
- Initial investigation suggests LVRS may benefit an expanded patient population, including carefully selected patients with homogenous emphysema and low DLCO.

INTRODUCTION: THE NATIONAL EMPHYSEMA TREATMENT TRIAL

Initial publication of the National Emphysema Treatment Trial (NETT) results in 2003 offered significant level I evidence in support of surgical therapy for the management of patients with severe emphysema.[1,2] This landmark prospective multicenter trial randomized a total of 1218 patients to either lung volume reduction surgery (LVRS) or medical management, marking a notable departure from the small, heterogeneous, single-center case series that comprised most of the existing data.[3–5] At the time of publication, NETT participants had a mean follow-up of 29 months and investigators reported on a range of outcomes including short- and long-term survival, maximal exercise performance, lung function, and quality of life.

Key study findings facilitated risk stratification and the ability to identify patients most likely to benefit from surgery. Based on 30-day surgical mortality, high-risk individuals were defined by forced expiratory volume in 1 second (FEV1) less than or equal to 20% predicted and a diffusion capacity for carbon monoxide (DLCO) less than or equal to 20% predicted, or a homogenous distribution of emphysema.[6] This subgroup was ultimately excluded from undergoing LVRS because they experienced an unacceptably high 30-day mortality rate of 16%. After removing these patients, statistically significant improvements in 6-minute-walk distance, FEV1% predicted, maximal exercise capacity, and disease-specific and general quality of life were found for non-high-risk patients who underwent LVRS as compared with medical therapy. Furthermore, in the subset of patients with upper-lobe-predominant emphysema and low exercise capacity, the surgery group had lower total mortality and improved exercise capacity and health-related quality of life at 24-month follow-up. Unfortunately, these benefits failed to persist for all study participants. Although patients with high exercise capacity did have a statistically significant improvement in exercise capacity and health-related quality of life, surgery

[a] Division of Cardiothoracic Surgery, Department of Surgery, University of Wisconsin-Madison, 600 Highland Avenue, Madison, WI 53792, USA; [b] Division of Cardiothoracic Surgery, University of Colorado, Anschutz Medical Campus, 12631 East 17th Avenue, Room 5401, Mail Stop C-291, Aurora, CO 80045, USA; [c] Division of Cardiothoracic Surgery, Department of Surgery, University of Wisconsin-Madison, 600 Highland Avenue, H4/340, Madison, WI 53792-0001, USA
* Corresponding author.
E-mail address: decamp@surgery.wisc.edu

Thorac Surg Clin 31 (2021) 119–128
https://doi.org/10.1016/j.thorsurg.2021.01.003

did not offer a survival benefit in this group. Furthermore, there was no surgical advantage in survival, exercise capacity, or health-related quality of life for patients with non-upper-lobe-predominant disease. In addition, analysis of postoperative outcomes suggested that only non-upper-lobe-predominant emphysema was predictive of increased operative mortality.

Aside from supplemental oxygen, LVRS is one of few available therapies proven to improve survival in select patients with emphysema. Together with updated results from 2006,[7] findings from NETT solidified surgery in the management algorithm of patients suffering from moderate to severe emphysema. Applying NETT inclusion and exclusion criteria to examine an academic medical center's pulmonary function laboratory database and radiology archive, Akuthota and colleagues[8] estimated 15% of emphysema patients could benefit from LVRS. Yet despite these data, widespread adoption of LVRS remains meager.[9] Although a precise rationale remains elusive, the cause of this marked underuse is likely multifactorial and includes limited access to approved surgical centers and pulmonary rehabilitation programs and confusion on behalf of medical providers regarding patient candidacy for surgery.[10] LVRS may also be falsely perceived as overly complicated and costly. Because NETT was a single payer (Centers for Medicare and Medicaid Services) trial, cost-effective analyses were feasible and enlightening. Using actual data from 3 and 5 years of clinical follow-up, NETT investigators showed Incremental Cost Effective Ratios for the upper-lobe-predominant emphysema patients that were comparable with Incremental Cost Effective Ratios used to support implantable defibrillators or heart transplantation. For example, the cost-effectiveness ratio for LVRS as compared with medical therapy for upper-lobe-predominant disease was reported as $77,000 per quality-adjusted life year gained at 5 years versus $65,0000 for heart transplantation.[11] More troubling, perhaps, is a misconception that the prohibitive postoperative outcomes from the high-risk group[6] apply more broadly to all patients with emphysema, creating a stigma of surgery as an excessively risky endeavor.

These fears have spurred innovation; recent years have seen development of less invasive means of lung volume reduction and important advancements in the understanding of disease characteristics and postoperative outcomes. In this article we highlight some of the salient research performed on LVRS published after the NETT in 2003, focusing on three important areas of investigation: (1) physiologic implications of LVRS, (2) recent data regarding the safety and durability of LVRS, and (3) patient selection and extension of NETT criteria to other patient populations.

PHYSIOLOGIC IMPLICATIONS OF LUNG VOLUME REDUCTION SURGERY

Lung volume reduction has proven effective in promoting enhanced exercise capacity, lung function, and quality of life for select patients with emphysema.[1,12] Although surgery was the first available means of volume reduction, less invasive strategies including endobronchial valves, coils, and sclerosing agents are under investigation.[13–15] Regardless of the technical execution, reducing lung volume is thought to combat the primary physiologic derangements of emphysema: airflow obstruction, asynchrony, and hyperinflation.[16] The primary mechanism was believed to be via increased elastic recoil pressure coupled with decreased airway resistance resultant from surgical resection of diseased lung.[17,18] In addition, resection of heterogenous lung parenchyma may counteract the effect of hyperinflation, providing decreased work of breathing and improved alveolar gas exchange.[19] However, recent investigation offers more sophisticated insight into the physiologic implications of lung volume reduction.

Emphysema results in diaphragmatic flattening, negatively impacting ventilatory mechanics through asynchronous chest movement and recruitment of abdominal musculature.[20] Furthermore, older studies suggest correlation between chest wall asynchrony, airflow obstruction, and breathlessness.[20,21] As such, Zoumot and colleagues[22] proposed improvements in chest wall asynchrony as an advantageous outcome of LVR. The authors conducted a single-institution prospective trial and randomized 26 patients under evaluation for LVR to either surgical or bronchoscopic LVR or sham treatment, using novel optoelectronic plethysmography generated three-dimensional volume measurements to assess chest wall asynchrony. Patients in the LVR group had statistically significant improvement in exercise capacity, quality of life, lung function, and radiographic evidence of decreased lung volume. The authors report high baseline levels of asynchrony in both groups. However, LVR patients had significantly greater improvement in asynchrony 3 months posttreatment, suggesting that this may correlate with symptomatic improvement.

Beyond asynchrony, recent investigation corroborates a long-term impact of LVRS on respiratory musculature. Using prospectively collected data from the NETT, Criner and colleagues[23] performed a retrospective analysis comparing pretreatment maximum inspiratory pressure (MIP) in patients who underwent LVRS versus medical management with MIP up to 36 months posttreatment. Patients in the LVRS group had significantly greater increase in MIP (19.8% compared with 3.2%) at 12 months. The improvement in MIP for patients who underwent LVRS peaked at 12 months but remained statistically significant at the 36-month follow-up. Male participants and those age 65 to 70 years had greater increase in MIP at all timepoints compared with their counterparts who received medical therapy. In accordance with original NETT findings, patients with upper-lobe-predominant disease and low exercise capacity also demonstrated sustained improvement in MIP at 24 months. The authors report an inverse relationship between MIP and noninvasive markers of dynamic hyperinflation, and propose that LVRS may promote clinical improvement by restoring optimal length-tension ratio of inspiratory musculature. This work builds on prior smaller studies suggesting a relationship between LVRS and improvement in MIP.[24,25]

Distinct from mechanical changes, LVRS may also impact inflammatory mediators associated with emphysema. Low-grade chronic inflammation likely plays an important role in the pathophysiology of emphysema; preponderance of leukocytes and deranged production of inflammatory mediators including increased tumor necrosis factor-α (TNF-α) and decreased α_1-antitrypsin (α_1-AT) have been reported.[26] With this in mind, Mineo and colleagues[27] proposed that LVRS reduced inflammatory mediators by removing emphysematous parenchyma. In a case-control study, the authors measured levels of inflammatory mediators and α_1-AT from 54 patients with severe emphysema (assigned to LVRS or standard respiratory rehabilitation program) and 25 healthy control subjects. Gene expression levels of protease-antiprotease and inflammatory mediators were also assessed from specimens in surgical patients. After 12 months, patients assigned to LVRS had significantly decreased levels of inflammatory mediators including TNF-α (-22.2%) and increased α_1-AT ($+27\%$) when compared with respiratory rehabilitation. Gene expression analysis revealed protease hyperactivity and predominant inflammation in diseased specimens, suggesting that surgery reduced the inflammatory burden by removing sites where these mediators were most heavily produced. Furthermore, study findings support a significant correlation between reduction in TNF-α, augmentation of α_1-AT, and decrease in residual volume (RV).

Better understanding of the relationship between LVRS, respiratory mechanics, and distribution of disease may improve the ability to select patients most likely to benefit from surgery. To this effect, Washko and colleagues[28] examined a subset of the NETT study population who underwent preoperative thoracic high-resolution computed tomographic (CT) scanning. Physiologic measures of lung recoil and inspiratory resistance were also measured but found not to be significantly associated with improvement in surgical outcomes, namely FEV1 or maximal exercise capacity after surgery. In contrast, preoperative CT assessment of the emphysema burden and ratio of upper to lower lobe disease demonstrated a weak, albeit statistically significant, association with improvement in FEV1 and exercise capacity postoperatively. Building on this foundation, recent radiographic advancements allow greater sophistication in quantifying the emphysema burden and distribution. An automated system can calculate the upper to lower zone ratio of low attenuation areas to facilitate selection of surgical candidates and target areas of resection. Although conventional CT remains the most commonly used radiographic assessment of surgical candidacy, dual-energy CT and dynamic MRI may offer important functional information to facilitate optional patient selection.[29,30]

EXAMINING SURGICAL SAFETY AND DURABILITY

Despite the NETT results demonstrating significant postoperative benefits and survival advantage for select patient populations, controversy persists regarding use of LVRS. Much of the debate stems from concern for unacceptably high surgical morbidity and mortality. Indeed, the 2003 NETT publication reported a sobering 90-day mortality of 5.5% for non-high-risk surgical patients compared with 1.5% following medical management.[1] This trepidation undoubtedly contributed to a marked decline in patients undergoing LVRS over the past decade in the United States and internationally.[31,32] However, long-term results from the original NETT publication and subsequent institutional data reinforce surgery as a safe treatment option in the setting of appropriate patient selection (**Table 1**).

In the wake of the initial NETT results, Naunheim and colleagues[7] published extended data in 2006, which included 40% more patients and two additional years of follow-up. This intention-to-treat study reinforced the overall survival benefit of surgery whereby the 5-year relative risk ratio for death was 0.86 (*P* = .02), with sustained improvements in

Table 1
Summary of outcomes following lung volume reduction surgery

Authors, Year of Publication	Study Design	Study Size	Procedural Morbidity and Mortality	Long-Term Outcomes
Naunheim et al,[7] 2006	Updated results from NETT (randomized controlled trial)	1218	5.5% 90-d mortality[1] 60% developed postoperative complication requiring intervention[38]	Upper-lobe-predominant low exercise capacity: 0.67 risk ratio for death at 5 y ($P = .003$) Symptom improvement at 5 y ($P = .01$) Exercise improvement at 3 y ($P<.001$)
Agzarian et al,[34] 2013	Retrospective observational analysis of patients randomized in the Canadian Lung Volume Reduction Surgery trial	62	0% 30-d surgical mortality Mortality at 2 y: 16% (LVRS) vs 13% (best medical care)[34]	Median survival 4.11 y 20% reduction in death rate compared with best medical care
Ginsburg et al,[36] 2016	Retrospective, single institution	91	0% 6-mo mortality 90% discharge to home Median length of stay 8 d	11% mean absolute increase in FEV1 at 5 y 4.1% increase in DLCO at 5 y 9.1 y median survival
van Agteren et al,[40] 2016	Meta-analysis	1760	Increased risk of postoperative death in short term (OR, 6.16; 95% CI, 3.22–11.79)	Decreased long-term mortality after surgery compared with medical care (OR, 0.76; 95% CI, 0.61–0.95)
Lim et al,[35] 2020	Re-evaluation of NETT data using longitudinal data methodology	1218	80.9% living independently 30 d after VATS LVRS[42]	At 5 y: 4.12 improvement in shortness of breath score ($P<.001$) 1.4% improvement in FEV1 ($P<.001$) 3.44% improvement in FVC ($P<.001$)

Abbreviations: CI, confidence interval; FVC, forced vital capacity; OR, odds ratio; VATS, video-assisted thoracoscopic surgery.

survival and symptoms at 5 years and exercise capacity at 3 years for patients with upper-lobe-predominant disease and low exercise capacity. These significant survival comparisons reflect a total mortality rate of 0.10 versus 0.12 deaths per person-year for patients treated surgically and medically, respectively. Furthermore, although the authors report no survival advantage for surgical patients with upper-lobe-predominant disease and high exercise capacity, these data support increased exercise capacity at 3 years and health-related quality of life at 4 years. Survival benefit was reinforced years later by the Canadian Lung Volume Reduction Surgery trial.[33] Subsequent publication of long-term follow-up results of this multicenter randomized controlled trial demonstrated superior median survival of 63 months in the surgery group compared with 47 months in patients receiving medical management.[34]

Recent work by Lim and colleagues[35] reinterpreted NETT data, positing that unclear presentation of clinical outcomes in the 2003 publication contributed to underuse of LVRS. Using longitudinal data analyses methodology, the authors aimed to re-examine lung function variables over time to provide conclusions on longer-term outcomes that were more readily interpretable to clinicians and patients. For surgical patients, FEV1 improved immediately postoperatively compared with medical therapy. The surgical advantage declined over time but was sustained after 5 years, at which point the residual difference was +1.47% of predicted (P<.001). Similarly, analysis of forced vital capacity and RV showed a small but sustained advantage in favor of LVRS at 5 years (+3.44%, −19.49%, respectively).

Impact on systemic physiologic function and symptom measures echoed the trajectory of lung function parameters. The authors report that patients randomized to LVRS had initial improvement in maximum workload capacity that declined over time but still favored surgery at 5 years. Similarly, improvements in shortness of breath and overall quality of well-being score for surgical patients persisted throughout the study period. The authors argue that patient-centered outcomes, such as quality of life and dyspnea, are more meaningful to patients and therefore may be used by clinicians to counsel those who are surgical candidates.

Since the Centers for Medicare and Medicaid Services approved the National Coverage Determination for LVRS in 2003, Ginsburg and colleagues[36] collected data on postoperative outcomes over a 10-year period. This single-institution retrospective study examined 91 patients who underwent bilateral LVRS between 2004 and 2014. Eighty-six percent of these patients received a bilateral video-assisted thoracoscopic surgery approach. All participants underwent comprehensive functional and radiographic evaluation, preoperative pulmonary rehabilitation, optimal medical therapy according to Global Initiative for Chronic Obstructive Lung Disease guidelines,[37] and were discussed at an interdisciplinary LVRS meeting to determine surgical candidacy before study enrollment. Selected patients met NETT criteria of having either upper-lobe-predominant disease and low exercise capacity or upper-lobe disease with high exercise capacity.

The authors report a 0% surgical mortality rate at 6 months. Patients spent an average of 8 days in the hospital after surgery, with 2 of those days in the intensive care unit. Remarkably, 90% of patients discharged directly home, and by the 6 month time point all patients were recovering at home. Three patients required reintubation or tracheostomy. The most common complication

was prolonged air leak lasting greater than 7 days (57%), with pneumonia (4%), cardiac arrhythmia (4%), and reoperation (3%) occurring with considerably less frequency. These outcomes are particularly striking when taken in comparison with original NETT results, which reported more than 20% of non-high-risk surgical patients required reintubation and fewer than 70% were able to return home 30 days postoperatively.[38,39]

Regarding treatment durability, the authors present favorable 1-, 2-, and 5-year functional results. Reported improvements in exercise capacity and lung function 1 and 2 years postoperatively echoed the 3-year post-NETT results from Naunheim and colleagues.[7] At 5 years, 24% and 36% of patients had sustained improvement in maximal workload and FEV1, respectively. These data reveal a median survival of 9.1 years and overall survival probability of 0.99 (95% confidence interval [CI], 0.96–1.00), 0.97 (95% CI, 0.93–1.00), and 0.78 (95% CI, 0.67–0.89) at 1, 2, and 5 years, respectively.

Recent Cochrane meta-analysis published in 2016 reviewed evidence from randomized-controlled trials comparing LVRS with nonsurgical treatment.[40] Authors identified 11 studies in total, which comprised a sum of 1760 patients. Key results included increased risk of death for patients undergoing LVRS in the short term (odds ratio, 6.16; 95% CI, 3.22–11.79). However, long-term mortality favored surgery (odds ratio, 0.76; 95% CI, 0.61–0.95). Moderate-quality evidence suggested surgical patients were more likely to demonstrate improvements in lung function parameters and quality of life as compared with control subjects, but this came at the price of higher treatment costs and adverse events including air leaks and cardiopulmonary morbidity.

It is worth acknowledging that significant advancements in surgical technique occurred since the original description of a lateral thoracotomy to resect emphysematous lung by Brantigan and coworkers in 1958.[41] The advent of video-assisted thoracoscopic surgery undoubtedly contributed to decreased surgical morbidity, yet this technique represented only 30% of patients in the NETT surgical cohort.[1] Within NETT, patients who underwent bilateral LVRS by video-assisted thoracoscopic surgery experienced morbidity and mortality comparable with those who received median sternotomy but had shorter intensive care unit stays and quicker overall recovery at reduced costs.[42] In addition, some have proposed a staged rather than the conventional simultaneous bilateral approach as an alternative strategy to reduce operative risk and improve long-term outcomes.[43] Oey and colleagues[43] conducted a comparative study suggesting improved functional improvements and 3- and 5-year survival regardless of operative timing. However, patients who underwent a staged approach had improved scores in health status questionnaires lasting up to 6 years.

BEYOND THE NATIONAL EMPHYSEMA TREATMENT TRIAL: EXTENDING SURGICAL CANDIDACY

The NETT clearly demonstrated that patients with heterogeneous upper-lobe-predominant disease and low exercise capacity responded best to LVRS[1]; these findings have been reinforced by subsequent investigation.[36] However, better understanding of disease physiology and the impact of surgery on respiratory mechanics have led investigators to push the boundaries of surgical candidacy.[44] Recent studies have explored outcomes of LVRS in patients with alternative disease morphology and pathology and the relationship between LVRS and lung transplantation.

Given that LVRS improves pulmonary mechanics through reduction of hyperinflated lung parenchyma, Weder and colleagues[45] hypothesized that this benefit would extend to patients with homogeneous emphysema. To test this, the authors selected 266 consecutive patients with severe emphysema who underwent bilateral LVRS and assessed disease distribution using CT and lung perfusion scintigraphy. The cohort of 138 patients with homogeneous disease demonstrated significant symptomatic and functional improvements at 3 months postoperatively. Specifically, FEV1 increased by 35% predicted and hyperinflation, as measured by the ratio of RV to total lung capacity, decreased by 15%. In addition, an increase in walking distance persisted for up to 2 years and dyspnea scores remained lower than baseline for up to 4 years. Although initial improvements were less pronounced compared with the heterogeneous emphysema cohort, duration of benefit was similar. Importantly, perioperative and 3 month mortality rates were similar between groups, suggesting that patients with homogeneous emphysema should not be categorically excluded from surgical therapy. In addition, recent investigation suggests volume reduction using endobronchial coils may provide similar benefit in the setting of severely hyperinflated homogeneous emphysema.[46]

Similarly, liberalizing the NETT criteria for DLCO and disease location has shown favorable results. In 33 patients with preoperative DLCO less than 20% and nonhomogeneous morphology, 90-day postoperative mortality was 0%.[44] In these patients the most common perioperative complication was prolonged air leak, occurring in nearly 50% of the cohort. Patients demonstrated significant improvement in median DLCO from 15% to 24% after surgery. Similarly, single-institutional data from the United Kingdom demonstrated improvement in FEV1 and ratio of RV to total lung capacity at 3 and 6 months postoperatively in 36 patients with lower-lobe-predominant disease.[47] Although these studies are undoubtedly small, nonrandomized investigations, they call into question the belief ingrained since the initial NETT publication that LVRS benefits only a small subset of patients with severe emphysema.

The role of LVRS for patients with α_1-AT disease has been less clear and previously overlooked. As such, Stoller and colleagues[48] analyzed outcomes of patients with α_1-AT disease within the NETT. Of 1218 patients, 1.3% were found to have severe α_1-AT disease. Ten of these patients underwent LVRS. In this small cohort, patients had decreased exercise capacity and shorter duration of improved FEV1 when compared with α_1-AT-replete individuals. Importantly, 2-year mortality was 20% and 0% in α_1-AT-deficient patients who underwent LVRS versus medical management, respectively, raising concern for use of surgical therapy in this population. More robust surgical data are unfortunately lacking; however, early investigation into the use of endobronchial coil treatment suggests more favorable results with significantly less procedural risk.[49]

Pulmonary hypertension was considered an absolute surgical contraindication in the NETT and this criteria persists in subsequent studies. However, newer data suggest that some of these patients may also benefit from surgery. Initial exclusion of patients with pulmonary hypertension was based on the theory that lung resection would exacerbate the condition because of anatomic reduction in the vascular bed. Yet, this anatomic alteration may be counteracted by decreased pulmonary vascular resistance from improved respiratory mechanics after LVRS.[50] Single-institution retrospective data from Switzerland reviewed 51 surgical patients who had undergone preoperative transthoracic echocardiography, 10 of whom had systolic pulmonary artery pressure greater than 35 mm Hg and heterogeneous emphysema.[51] The authors report 0% 90-day mortality in the pulmonary hypertension group and median systolic pulmonary artery pressure decreased from 41 mm Hg to 37 mm Hg. Significant improvements in FEV1% predicted and hyperinflation were also noted. Subsequent investigation from the United States compared in-hospital and 1-year outcomes in 124 patients who underwent LVRS.[52] In the 56 patients with pulmonary hypertension (defined by mean systolic pulmonary artery pressure greater than 35 mm Hg on right heart catheterization), the authors report no significant difference in hours of mechanical ventilation, intensive care days, prolonged air leak, or hospital length of stay when compared with patients without pulmonary hypertension. Furthermore, functional outcomes and quality-of-life scores were similar between groups at 1 year. Despite these encouraging findings, current evidence is limited to small retrospective analyses causing some to favor lung transplant over LVRS in this patient population.[53] Surgical management should proceed with caution; analysis of lung transplant following LVRS found severe pulmonary hypertension to be a significant risk factor for post-transplant mortality.[54]

Both LVRS and lung transplantation represent potential treatment options for patients with end-stage emphysema. Deciding between surgical treatment options requires careful consideration of complex clinical and social factors catered to the individual patient.[53] Retrospective analysis conducted by Weinstein and colleagues[55] offers a head-to-head comparison of these surgical therapies. One year following surgery, transplant patients had statistically significant improvement in FEV1% predicted (43.4% vs 2.2%) and modified BODE index (−5.7 vs −2.0) when compared with LVRS. However, this came at the cost of lower long-term survival and greater mean total costs. Not surprisingly, transplant patients spent more time in the hospital and required more frequent outpatient follow-up.

In addition to stand-alone therapy, LVRS may be considered as a strategy to delay transplant listing or as a bridge to transplant; however, the data remain mixed.[56] Contemporary analysis raised concerns regarding inferior graft function and increased postoperative complications in patients who were transplanted following LVRS.[54] In addition, work by Backhus and colleagues[57] revealed inferior post-transplant survival associated with transplant following LVRS. Although 30-day mortality was similar between groups, median post-transplant survival diverged in favor of transplant alone (49 months vs 96 months for transplant following LVRS and transplant alone, respectively). The authors attribute this discrepancy at least in part to increased operative times and hospital length of stay associated with transplantation after LVRS. Post-LVRS survival was equivalent regardless of whether the patient went on to receive a transplant, which may speak to the role of transplantation in extending lifespan in more severely ill patients following LVRS. These findings are in contrast with a recent report from the Registry of the International Society for Heart and Lung Transplantation,

which demonstrates similar 1- and 5-year survival regardless of surgical approach.[58] Similarly, single-institution survival analysis of patients undergoing lung transplant between 1993 and 2014 reported 10% in-hospital mortality, which was unrelated to prior receipt of LVRS. Furthermore, improved median survival trended in favor of transplant following LVRS (107 vs 86 months) but this was not statistically significant.[59]

SUMMARY

Since publication of the initial findings of the NETT in 2003, great strides have been made in the understanding and provision of surgical treatment of patients with moderate and severe emphysema. Greater sophistication of surgical technique and deeper insight into the physiologic implications of lung volume reduction have paved the way for improved outcomes and innovative therapeutic alternatives. These findings have important implications for surgeons, researchers, and patients.

For researchers, increased understanding of the mechanisms by which volume reduction alters pulmonary mechanics to enact meaningful clinical benefit facilitates development of less invasive treatments. Significant work is already underway in the development and testing of endobronchial valves and coils that portend symptomatic improvement with less morbidity than surgery.[13,15] Furthermore, technological advancements in preoperative imaging offer enhanced precision in patient selection for surgery.

For surgeons, recent investigation reinforces the benefit and durability of LVRS. Institutional data suggesting operative 6-month mortality rates of 0% with a favorable morbidity profile[36] and functional improvements extending to 5 years postoperatively[7,35] may aid in reversing the nihilism regarding surgery that contributed to underuse. Early exploration into expanded patient eligibility, particularly in terms of homogeneous disease distribution and pulmonary hypertension, should encourage surgeons to evaluate each patient individually before determining candidacy for surgery.

Finally, and most importantly, recent literature suggests that surgery may offer patients with emphysema the opportunity for improved quality of life, pulmonary function, and overall survival. These benefits may be achieved at a lesser cost in terms of morbidity and mortality and be applicable to a broader selection of patients than previously thought. Recent data regarding surgical risks and longer-term outcomes may facilitate preoperative counseling to ensure that patients enter a treatment pathway with a better understanding of the implications of surgery.

CLINICS CARE POINT

- In appropriately selected patients, bilateral LVRS provides durable physiologic, functional and quality-of-life benefits which exceed those achieved with best medical therapy.

DISCLOSURE

Dr D.P. McCarthy receives research support from Ethicon Inc and Intuitive Surgical. Dr L.J. Taylor and Dr M.M. DeCamp do not have any commercial or financial conflicts of interest.

REFERENCES

1. Fishman A, Martinez F, Naunheim K, et al. A randomized trial comparing lung-volume-reduction surgery with medical therapy for severe emphysema. N Engl J Med 2003;348(21):2059–73.
2. Concato J, Shah N, Horwitz RI. Randomized, controlled trials, observational studies, and the hierarchy of research designs. N Engl J Med 2000; 342(25):1887–92.
3. Bingisser R, Zollinger A, Hauser M, et al. Bilateral volume reduction surgery for diffuse pulmonary emphysema by video-assisted thoracoscopy. J Thorac Cardiovasc Surg 1996;112(4):875–82.
4. Cooper JD, Patterson GA, Sundaresan RS, et al. Results of 150 consecutive bilateral lung volume reduction procedures in patients with severe emphysema. J Thorac Cardiovasc Surg 1996;112(5):1319–29 [discussion 1329–30].
5. Daniel TM, Chan BB, Bhaskar V, et al. Lung volume reduction surgery. Case selection, operative technique, and clinical results. Ann Surg 1996;223(5): 526–31 [discussion: 532–3].
6. Patients at high risk of death after lung-volume–reduction surgery. N Engl J Med 2001;345(15): 1075–83.
7. Naunheim KS, Wood DE, Mohsenifar Z, et al. Long-term follow-up of patients receiving lung-volume-reduction surgery versus medical therapy for severe emphysema by the National Emphysema Treatment Trial Research Group. Ann Thorac Surg 2006;82(2): 431–43.
8. Akuthota P, Litmanovich D, Zutler M, et al. An evidence-based estimate on the size of the potential patient pool for lung volume reduction surgery. Ann Thorac Surg 2012;94(1):205–11.
9. Decker MR, Leverson GE, Jaoude WA, et al. Lung volume reduction surgery since the National Emphysema Treatment Trial: study of Society of Thoracic Surgeons Database. J Thorac Cardiovasc Surg 2014;148(6):2651–8.e1.
10. Criner GJ, Cordova F, Sternberg AL, et al. The National Emphysema Treatment Trial (NETT) part II: lessons learned about lung volume reduction surgery. Am J Respir Crit Care Med 2011;184(8):881–93.
11. Ramsey SD, Sullivan SD, Kaplan RM. Cost-effectiveness of lung volume reduction surgery. Proc Am Thorac Soc 2008;5(4):406–11.
12. van Geffen WH, Slebos DJ, Herth FJ, et al. Surgical and endoscopic interventions that reduce lung volume for emphysema: a systemic review and meta-analysis. Lancet Respir Med 2019;7(4):313–24.
13. Criner GJ, Sue R, Wright S, et al. A multicenter randomized controlled trial of zephyr endobronchial valve treatment in heterogeneous emphysema (LIBERATE). Am J Respir Crit Care Med 2018; 198(9):1151–64.
14. Criner GJ, Delage A, Voelker K, et al. Improving lung function in severe heterogenous emphysema with the spiration valve system (EMPROVE). a multicenter, open-label randomized controlled clinical trial. Am J Respir Crit Care Med 2019;200(11): 1354–62.
15. Sciurba FC, Criner GJ, Strange C, et al. Effect of Endobronchial Coils vs usual care on exercise tolerance in patients with severe emphysema: the RENEW randomized clinical trial. JAMA 2016; 315(20):2178–89.
16. Brenner M, Yusen R, McKenna R Jr, et al. Lung volume reduction surgery for emphysema. Chest 1996; 110(1):205–18.
17. Gelb AF, Gold WM, Wright RR, et al. Physiologic diagnosis of subclinical emphysema. Am Rev Respir Dis 1973;107(1):50–63.
18. Rogers RM, DuBois AB, Blakemore WS. Effect of removal of bullae on airway conductance and conductance volume ratios. J Clin Invest 1968; 47(12):2569–79.
19. Fessler HE, Scharf SM, Ingenito EP, et al. Physiologic basis for improved pulmonary function after lung volume reduction. Proc Am Thorac Soc 2008; 5(4):416–20.
20. Gilmartin JJ, Gibson GJ. Abnormalities of chest wall motion in patients with chronic airflow obstruction. Thorax 1984;39(4):264–71.
21. Celli BR, Rassulo J, Make BJ. Dyssynchronous breathing during arm but not leg exercise in patients with chronic airflow obstruction. N Engl J Med 1986; 314(23):1485–90.
22. Zoumot Z, LoMauro A, Aliverti A, et al. Lung volume reduction in emphysema improves chest wall asynchrony. Chest 2015;148(1):185–95.
23. Criner RN, Yu D, Jacobs MR, et al. Effect of lung volume reduction surgery on respiratory muscle strength in advanced emphysema. Chronic Obstr Pulm Dis 2018;6(1):40–50.
24. Martinez FJ, de Oca MM, Whyte RI, et al. Lung-volume reduction improves dyspnea, dynamic

hyperinflation, and respiratory muscle function. Am J Respir Crit Care Med 1997;155(6):1984–90.

25. Criner G, Cordova FC, Leyenson V, et al. Effect of lung volume reduction surgery on diaphragm strength. Am J Respir Crit Care Med 1998;157(5 Pt 1):1578–85.

26. Barnes PJ. Chronic obstructive pulmonary disease. N Engl J Med 2000;343(4):269–80.

27. Mineo D, Ambrogi V, Cufari ME, et al. Variations of inflammatory mediators and alpha1-antitrypsin levels after lung volume reduction surgery for emphysema. Am J Respir Crit Care Med 2010; 181(8):806–14.

28. Washko GR, Martinez FJ, Hoffman EA, et al. Physiological and computed tomographic predictors of outcome from lung volume reduction surgery. Am J Respir Crit Care Med 2010;181(5):494–500.

29. Martini K, Frauenfelder T. Emphysema and lung volume reduction: the role of radiology. J Thorac Dis 2018;10(Suppl 23):S2719–31.

30. Martini K, Caviezel C, Schneiter D, et al. Dynamic magnetic resonance imaging as an outcome predictor for lung-volume reduction surgery in patients with severe emphysema†. Eur J Cardiothorac Surg 2019; 55(3):446–54.

31. Marchetti N, Criner GJ. Surgical approaches to treating emphysema: lung volume reduction surgery, bullectomy, and lung transplantation. Semin Respir Crit Care Med 2015;36(4):592–608.

32. Whittaker HR, Connell O, Campbell J, et al. Eligibility for lung volume reduction surgery in patients with COPD identified in a UK primary care setting. Chest 2020;157(2):276–85.

33. Miller JD, Malthaner RA, Goldsmith CH, et al. A randomized clinical trial of lung volume reduction surgery versus best medical care for patients with advanced emphysema: a two-year study from Canada. Ann Thorac Surg 2006;81(1):314–20 [discussion: 320–1].

34. Agzarian J, Miller JD, Kosa SD, et al. Long-term survival analysis of the Canadian Lung Volume Reduction Surgery trial. Ann Thorac Surg 2013;96(4): 1217–22.

35. Lim E, Sousa I, Shah PL, et al. Lung volume reduction surgery: reinterpreted with longitudinal data analyses methodology. Ann Thorac Surg 2020;109(5): 1496–501.

36. Ginsburg ME, Thomashow BM, Bulman WA, et al. The safety, efficacy, and durability of lung-volume reduction surgery: a 10-year experience. J Thorac Cardiovasc Surg 2016;151(3):717–24.e1.

37. Vestbo J, Hurd SS, Agustí AG, et al. Global strategy for the diagnosis, management, and prevention of chronic obstructive pulmonary disease: GOLD executive summary. Am J Respir Crit Care Med 2013;187(4):347–65.

38. DeCamp MM Jr, McKenna RJ Jr, Deschamps CC, et al. Lung volume reduction surgery: technique, operative mortality, and morbidity. Proc Am Thorac Soc 2008;5(4):442–6.

39. Criner GJ, Sternberg AL. National emphysema treatment trial: the major outcomes of lung volume reduction surgery in severe emphysema. Proc Am Thorac Soc 2008;5(4):393–405.

40. van Agteren JE, Carson KV, Tiong LU, et al. Lung volume reduction surgery for diffuse emphysema. Cochrane Database Syst Rev 2016;(10):CD001001.

41. Brantigan OC, Mueller E, Kress MB. A surgical approach to pulmonary emphysema. Am Rev Respir Dis 1959;80(1, Part 2):194–206.

42. McKenna RJ Jr, Benditt JO, DeCamp M, et al. Safety and efficacy of median sternotomy versus video-assisted thoracic surgery for lung volume reduction surgery. J Thorac Cardiovasc Surg 2004;127(5): 1350–60.

43. Oey IF, Morgan MD, Spyt TJ, et al. Staged bilateral lung volume reduction surgery - the benefits of a patient-led strategy. Eur J Cardiothorac Surg 2010; 37(4):846–52.

44. Caviezel C, Schneiter D, Opitz I, et al. Lung volume reduction surgery beyond the NETT selection criteria. J Thorac Dis 2018;10(Suppl 23):S2748–53.

45. Weder W, Tutic M, Lardinois D, et al. Persistent benefit from lung volume reduction surgery in patients with homogeneous emphysema. Ann Thorac Surg 2009;87(1):229–36 [discussion: 236–7].

46. Marchetti N, Kaufman T, Chandra D, et al. Endobronchial Coils versus lung volume reduction surgery or medical therapy for treatment of advanced homogenous emphysema. Chronic Obstr Pulm Dis 2018;5(2):87–96.

47. Perikleous P, Sharkey A, Oey I, et al. Long-term survival and symptomatic relief in lower lobe lung volume reduction surgery. Eur J Cardiothorac Surg 2017;52(5):982–8.

48. Stoller JK, Gildea TR, Ries AL, et al. Lung volume reduction surgery in patients with emphysema and alpha-1 antitrypsin deficiency. Ann Thorac Surg 2007;83(1):241–51.

49. Perotin JM, Leroy S, Marquette CH, et al. Endobronchial coil treatment in severe emphysema patients with alpha-1 antitrypsin deficiency. Int J Chron Obstruct Pulmon Dis 2018;13:3645–9.

50. Opitz I, Ulrich S. Pulmonary hypertension in chronic obstructive pulmonary disease and emphysema patients: prevalence, therapeutic options and pulmonary circulatory effects of lung volume reduction surgery. J Thorac Dis 2018;10(Suppl 23):S2763–74.

51. Caviezel C, Aruldas C, Franzen D, et al. Lung volume reduction surgery in selected patients with emphysema and pulmonary hypertension. Eur J Cardiothorac Surg 2018;54(3):565–71.

52. Thuppal S, Crabtree T, Markwell S, et al. Pulmonary hypertension: a contraindication for lung volume reduction surgery? Ann Thorac Surg 2020;109(3): 902–6.

53. Patel N, DeCamp M, Criner GJ. Lung transplantation and lung volume reduction surgery versus transplantation in chronic obstructive pulmonary disease. Proc Am Thorac Soc 2008;5(4):447–53.

54. Shigemura N, Gilbert S, Bhama JK, et al. Lung transplantation after lung volume reduction surgery. Transplantation 2013;96(4):421–5.

55. Weinstein MS, Martin UJ, Crookshank AD, et al. Mortality and functional performance in severe emphysema after lung volume reduction or transplant. COPD 2007;4(1):15–22.

56. Slama A, Taube C, Kamler M, et al. Lung volume reduction followed by lung transplantation-considerations on selection criteria and outcome. J Thorac Dis 2018;10(Suppl 27):S3366–75.

57. Backhus L, Sargent J, Cheng A, et al. Outcomes in lung transplantation after previous lung volume reduction surgery in a contemporary cohort. J Thorac Cardiovasc Surg 2014;147(5):1678–83.e1.

58. Chambers DC, Yusen RD, Cherikh WS, et al. The registry of the International Society for Heart and Lung Transplantation: thirty-fourth adult lung and heart-lung transplantation report-2017; focus theme: allograft ischemic time. J Heart Lung Transplant 2017;36(10):1047–59.

59. Inci I, Iskender I, Ehrsam J, et al. Previous lung volume reduction surgery does not negatively affect survival after lung transplantation. Eur J Cardiothorac Surg 2018;53(3):596–602.

Technical Aspects of Lung Volume Reduction Surgery Including Anesthetic Management and Surgical Approaches

Philippe H. Lemaitre, MD, PhD, Bryan Payne Stanifer, MD, MPH, Joshua R. Sonett, MD, Mark E. Ginsburg, MD*

KEYWORDS

• LVRS • Minimally invasive thoracic surgery • Subxiphoid

KEY POINTS

• Lung volume reduction surgery (LVRS) can be offered to a carefully selected subset of chronic obstructive pulmonary disease patients.
• Bilateral LVRS is recommended.
• Minimally invasive approaches improve outcomes.
• Extrathoracic subxiphoid incision with subcostal ports decrease postoperative pain to improve spontaneous breathing and early mobilization.

INTRODUCTION

Initially described in the 1950s by Brantigan and colleagues,[1] lung volume reduction surgery (LVRS) was highly controversial until the completion of the National Emphysema Treatment Trial (NETT) in the late 1990s.[2] This study demonstrated that patients with both upper-lobe predominant emphysema and low baseline exercise capacity benefited from surgery in terms of survival and quality of life. It also demonstrated this benefit was durable.[2] Patients assigned to LVRS in the NETT underwent bilateral stapled lung volume reduction through either a median sternotomy (MS) or a video-assisted bilateral thoracic surgery (VATS). With stringent selection criteria being adopted after the NETT trial, the subsequent era saw a transition from maximally invasive resections carried out via sternotomy toward bilateral VATS surgeries. For these procedures, the intraoperative general anesthesia was complemented by an epidural catheter to improve postoperative pain management and allow for early patient mobilization. In this article, the authors review the historical evolution of surgical techniques used to perform LVRS, including the recent development of subxiphoid surgery, especially when coupled with subcostal port placement further reduced postoperative pain.

ANESTHETIC MANAGEMENT

LVRS is routinely performed under intubated general anesthesia using a left-sided double-lumen endotracheal tube (ET). A single lumen tube can first be placed to perform flexible bronchoscopy for evaluation of the bronchial tree and to assess and clear secretions. A microbiology sample should be obtained to help guide antibiotic management should the patient develop postoperative infectious complications.

Department of Thoracic Surgery, NewYork-Presbyterian Columbia University Irving Medical Center, Herbert Irving Pavilion, 161 Fort Washington Avenue, 3rd Floor, New York, NY 10032, USA
* Corresponding author.
E-mail address: meg18@cumc.columbia.edu

Thorac Surg Clin 31 (2021) 129–137
https://doi.org/10.1016/j.thorsurg.2021.02.001
1547-4127/21/© 2021 Elsevier Inc. All rights reserved.

Ventilation must be protective during surgery, as the major risk faced by chronic obstructive pulmonary disease (COPD) patients during positive pressure ventilation is a further increase in air trapping resulting in hemodynamic instability. Low tidal volumes (5–8 mL/kg) to achieve low plateau pressures (<15–20 cm H_2O) and low to no positive end-expiratory pressure at a slower rate (10–12 breaths per minute) to increase in the inspiratory-to-expiratory ratio (1:3) are strategies to prevent air trapping. Nevertheless, disconnecting the ET from the vent will drop ventilator tension-related life-threatening situations. If the patient remains hypotensive upon ET tube disconnection, the alternative diagnosis of tension pneumothorax must be evoked and addressed. Soon after positioning, ventilation to the first addressed side must be stopped to allow enough time for the lung to deflate.

The major downside of protective ventilation in these patients is hypercapnia, which will be tolerated in a "permissive" strategy as long as pH is kept greater than 7.25. This permissive strategy also includes oxygenation, as Fio_2 is kept as low as possible to achieve saturations greater than 90%. Before extubation, the permissive hypercapnia must be recognized and fully reversed to avoid and exacerbate the drowsiness associated with higher $Paco_2$ after extubation. For the same purpose, the authors very cautiously use opioids for pain management during LVRS, as their undesirable effects (eg, prolonged respiratory depression) may greatly impact the early postoperative period. Short-acting synthetic opioids (eg, fentanyl or remifentanil) are therefore definitively preferred intraoperatively in these patients.[3] Opioids should be used very cautiously postoperatively and avoided in the epidural in the early postoperative period.

Over time, refinements in the authors' surgical techniques have resulted in less surgical pain, which, on the one hand, decreases pain management requirements, and on the other hand, improves early patient mobilization postoperatively. By using the fully extrathoracic approach depicted in later discussion, the authors have now moved away from using epidural catheters in LVRS patients. Ultimately, the goal is to improve the patient's respiratory drive after extubation and in the early postoperative period. Extubated, awake, and alert patients are then transferred to the intensive care unit (ICU) for 24 to 48 hours of monitoring. Patients failing this strategy are placed on bilevel positive airway pressure (BiPAP) or continuous positive airway pressure (CPAP). The authors favor early tracheostomy for patients who are finally reintubated.

SURGICAL ASPECTS
Strategy

Following the NETT trial and with experience, more data concerning LVRS became available, defining inclusion and exclusion criteria for LVRS. Patient selection is the initial step of the surgical strategy, and these patient characteristics have been shown to accurately predict outcome. The authors therefore recommend diligently respecting these criteria as a critical guide to develop a safe LVRS program[4] (**Table 1**). Next, although unilateral LVRS may produce an excellent result in the highly selected patient, the bilateral procedure has been shown to be the procedure of choice, because it provides improved survival and physiology with no increased morbidity or mortality compared with the unilateral procedure[5] (**Table 2**).

Even if unilateral procedures are staged to yield a bilateral result, the cost of 2 operations and hospitalizations have never been justified.[5] The authors currently always perform bilateral procedures outside of considerations that preclude them from operating on the other side.[6] Conditions allwoing to consider unilateral LVRS include include the rare purely unilateral disease, contralateral pleurodesis, or previous thoracotomy; hemodynamic instability during single-lung ventilation; massive air leaks after first-side LVRS; or contralateral lung transplantation with native lung hyperinflation. It should be noted that prior thoracotomy is not an absolute contraindication to LVRS and can be safely performed under strict guidelines.

The goal of LVRS is to resect by peripheral resection 25% to 35% of the ipsilateral lung volume of the most emphysematous portions of the diseased lung. In most forms of emphysema, destructed areas reside within the upper lobes. Resection targets can be identified preoperatively by perfusion scans and computed tomographic scanning and confirmed by intraoperative observations. Intraoperative lung targeting is performed using the following techniques: (1) the more normal lung retains its elastic recoil and becomes atelectatic faster upon stopping lung ventilation, whereas the more diseased areas become atelectatic more slowly or not at all; (2) more normal lung loses its perfusion during atelectasis and becomes cyanotic, whereas the more emphysematous lung remains pink; (3) reventilating the atelectatic lung results in reexpansion of the more diseased lung first.

Over several decades of performing LVRS, the authors have learned to progressively abandon very aggressive resections and to try to tailor the remaining lung to fill the thoracic cage, still reducing lung volume sufficiently to achieve

Table 1
Inclusion and exclusion criteria for selecting patients for lung volume reduction surgery

Inclusion Criteria	Exclusion Criteria
History and physical examination, chest roentgenogram, and HRCT scan consistent with bilateral emphysema	CT evidence of diffuse emphysema judged inappropriate for LVRS
Severe upper-lobe predominant emphysema	Dysrhythmia or exercise-related syncope that might pose a risk during exercise or training
Severe non-upper-lobe predominant emphysema with low exercise capacity	Resting bradycardia; frequent multifocal PVCs; complex ventricular arrhythmia; sustained SVT
Body mass index $\leq$31.1 kg/m^2 (men) or $\leq$32.3 kg/m^2 (women)	Myocardial infarction within 6 mo and LVEF <45%
Stable with $\leq$20 mg prednisone (or equivalent) each day	Congestive heart failure within 6 mo and LVEF <45%
Plasma cotinine level $\leq$13.7 ng/mL (or arterial carboxyhemoglobin $\leq$2.5% if using nicotine products)	Uncontrolled hypertension (systolic >200 mm; diastolic >110 mm)
Non-smoking for 4 mo	History of recurrent infections with clinically significant sputum production
FEV1 $\geq$45% predicted (15% predicted if age 70 y)	Pleural or interstitial disease that precludes surgery
TLC $\geq$100% predicted postbronchodilator	Clinically significant bronchiectasis
RV $\geq$150% predicted postbronchodilator	Previous lung transplant, LVRS, lobectomy
P_{CO_2} $\leq$60 mm Hg	Pulmonary hypertension: peak systolic PAP $\geq$45 mm Hg or mean PAP $\geq$35 mm Hg
P_{O_2} $\geq$45 mm Hg on room air	Requirement for > 6 L oxygen to keep saturation $\geq$90% with exercise
Postrehabilitation 6-min walk distance of $\geq$140 m	Unplanned weight loss of >10% usual weight in previous 90 d
Able to complete 3 min unloaded pedaling in exercise tolerance test	
Approval for surgery by cardiologist if unstable angina, LVEF <45%, arrhythmia	

Abbreviations: CT, computed tomography; FEV1, forced expiratory volume in 1 second; HRCT, high-resolution computed tomography; LVEF, left ventricular ejection fraction; PAP, pulmonary arterial pressure; PVC, premature ventricular contraction; RV, residual volume; SVT, supraventricular tachycardia; TLC, total lung capacity.
From Seadler B, Thuppal S, Rizvi N, et al. Clinical and Quality of Life Outcomes After Lung Volume Reduction Surgery. Ann. Thorac. Surg 2019;108: 866-872; with permission.

adequate physiologic improvement in ventilation. In the early days of LVRS, overresection resulted in large residual airspaces that predisposed to prolonged and difficult to manage air leaks for a disputable functional benefit. Overresection undoubtedly contributed to the high morbidity and mortality that occurred in the pre-NETT and NETT period. The goal of LVRS is to adequately reduce volume, not to remove all of the diseased lung. Of note, disease can also affect the lower lobes, especially in the context of alpha-1 antitrypsin deficiency, and surgery can be offered in this context with decent outcomes.[7,8]

Although bilateral LVRS was initially carried out via bilateral thoracotomies by Brantigan, Cooper and colleagues[9,10] used MS for this procedure. A less aggressive thoracic approach, VATS, became popular in the 1990s and quickly appeared quite ideally suited for LVRS. With experience, it was shown that VATS LVRS allowed earlier recovery at a lower cost than MS, possibly because of reduced surgical trauma from a minimally invasive surgery.[5,11–13] In the authors' experience, they have performed all LVRS using VATS approaches since 2005.

Last, postoperative management is the closing critical aspect in LVRS. The authors still use an

Table 2
Unilateral versus bilateral lung volume reduction surgery outcomes

Author, Year	n	Technique	Mortality (%)	LOS (d)	Change in FEV$_1$
McKenna,[8] 1996	87	Unilateral	3	11.4	31%
Naunheim,[7] 1996	50	Unilateral	2	13	35%
Keenan,[9] 1996	57	Unilateral	2	17	27%
Cooper,[10] 1996	150	Bilateral	4	13.5	51%
Kotloff,[4] 1996	80	Bilateral	13.8	22	41%
Argentano,[5] 1996	85	Bilateral	7	17	61%
McKenna,[11] 1997	154	Bilateral	4	11	52%
Kotloff,[4] 1996	40	Bilateral	2. S	15	41%
NETT,[18,19] 2003/4	511	Bilateral	2.2	10	NR

Abbreviations: LOS, length of stay; NR, not reported.
From DeCamp MM, Jr., McKenna RJ, Jr., Deschamps CC, Krasna MJ. 2008. Lung volume reduction surgery: technique, operative mortality, and morbidity. *Proc Am Thorac Soc.* Vol 5(4):442-446.

ICU environment for their initial postoperative period but with early mobilization. Every attempt is made to extubate the patient in the operating room, and this has been successful routinely in the post-NETT era. The authors recommend aggressive incentive spirometry, physiotherapy, and mobilization as soon as the patient's clinical condition allows. Chest tubes are connected to low suction until the authors can safely transition to water seal. Pain management is critical, and balancing opioid use with CO_2 levels is important. BiPAP or CPAP can be helpful for the marginal patient to help carry them through the early postoperative period. Awake bronchoscopy for secretions can be helpful in the occasional patient not responding to physiotherapy, suctioning, and steroids. In the face of prolonged air leaks, the authors discharge patients home as soon as they can be safely connected to a Heimlich valve.

The Lateral Video-Assisted Bilateral Thoracic Surgery Approach

The early yet most currently used VATS procedure to achieve bilateral LVRS is to perform 2 lateral approaches starting with the most diseased side. As most surgeons, the authors prefer to position the patient supine with the arms above the head and strapped to a padded bar (**Fig. 1**). Blanket rolls placed under the shoulders, hips, and along the spine, or a beanbag, elevate the patient off the operative table to provide more lateral port access. Such positioning avoids the need to reposition and redrape the patient for 2 sequential lateral approaches, which improves surgical efficiency and cost-effectiveness of the procedure and allows for an easy access to the contralateral side in the face of complications.

Technically, the lateral video-assisted bilateral thoracic surgery (LVATS) procedure can be carried out using either 3 ports, 1 port and 1 utility incision, or 1 working incision alone. In general, ports or incisions should be placed as anterior as possible to take advantage of the wider intercostal interspaces on the anterior chest wall, thus decreasing torsion injury to the intercostal nerves and postoperative pain. Port placement posterior to the scapula should therefore be avoided. All sites are preemptively locally injected with a solution of bupivacaine 0.25% with epinephrine 1:200,000 (Sensorcaine; Fresenius Kabi, Lake Zurich, IL, USA), which enhances pain control and reduces the nuisance of blood dribbling from the ports during the surgery.

For a 3-incision approach, the chest is usually entered with a 5-mm port placed in the eighth intercostal space on the anterior axillary line, and a 30-degree angled camera is used to place the other ports under direct vision. The authors then place a 12-mm port anteriorly in the sixth intercostal space, as this location offers the widest space to accommodate such larger "stapler" port. Last, the triangle is completed by placing a second 5-mm port in the seventh or eighth intercostal space more posteriorly. When using only 2 incisions, a 5-cm utility incision can be placed in the fifth intercostal space just anterior to the anterior axillary line. The authors use a small Alexis O-Ring (Applied Medical, Rancho Santa Margarita, CA, USA) to keep this access open. For the uniportal procedure, only the fifth intercostal space incision is used (**Fig. 2**).

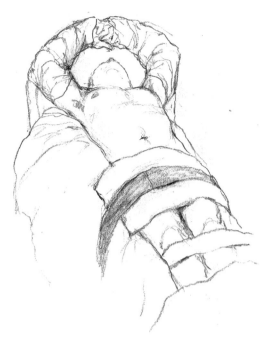

Fig. 1. Patient positioning with arms above the head and padding. The patient is positioned supine with the arms above the head and strapped to a padded bar. Blanket rolls placed under the shoulders, hips, and along the spine, or a beanbag, elevate the patient off the operative table to provide more lateral port access. (*Courtesy of* Linda Capello, Sag Harbor, New York, USA.)

The LVATS approach offers great benefit in that it replicates the exact same visual orientation as that of open surgery. Less-experienced surgeons will therefore find it comforting to use. Following port placement, the pleural cavity is fully explored to rule out any condition that could prevent proceeding. Adhesions are taken down if needed using gentle dissection, as this maneuver is a definitive risk factor for air leaks. Use of CO_2 can at times substantially improve exposure, and the extrapleural route can be used in unsafe areas. When carrying out these dissections, the authors cannot emphasize enough the importance of avoiding the phrenic nerve injury, as this is an even more dreadful complication in LVRS than in other thoracic conditions. It can therefore be helpful to divide the lung first, then dissect adhesions, or even leave a rim of lung attached to the phrenic area. Of note, surgical judgment regarding adherences is critical. The goal is to allow the healthy lung to expand and slide to fill the pleural cavity; this requires the freeing of all adherences.

When the lung is completely mobilized and free, the visual difference between atelectatic healthy and the still inflated diseased lung together with the preoperative imaging-based LVRS plan allow

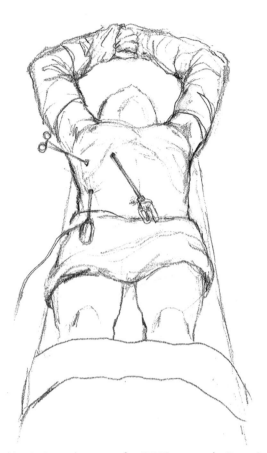

Fig. 2. Port placement for LVATS approach. For a 3-incision approach, the chest is entered with a 5-mm port placed in the eighth intercostal space on the anterior axillary line, and a 30-degree angled camera is used to place the other ports under direct vision. The second port (12 mm) is placed anteriorly in the sixth intercostal space. The third port (5 mm) is placed in the seventh or eighth intercostal space more posteriorly. (*Courtesy of* Linda Capello, Sag Harbor, New York, USA.)

identification of the diseased areas. Manipulating these fragile areas is prone to tearing and must therefore be avoided. In this perspective, the authors first recommend operating on a deflated lung, which can be rapidly accomplished by using the cautery to fenestrate the most bullous areas: the marked collateral ventilation leads to prompt collapse. Next, the authors recommend grasping exclusively the diseased areas that will then be resected.

The NETT trial mandated a bilateral stapled approach to LVRS.[14] Initially designed for bowel resections, staplers evolved over time and are nowadays the most common way to divide the lung. Specifically, buttressed staple lines became popular for LVRS following early reports showing reduced air leaks, even if this idea was subsequently challenged.[15–17]

The authors currently use linear polyglycolic acid buttressed staplers (Endo GIA Reinforced Reload with Tri-Staple technology; Medtronic, Minneapolis, MN, USA) with the addition of surgical glues as sealants at the discretion of the surgeon. Other buttressing compounds include strips of bovine pericardium or polytetrafluoroethylene, but the material does not seem to affect aerostasis.

The staple line is created from anterior to posterior. On the right side, the authors start straight across the middle lobe beginning medially above the hilum and ending up just above the posterior aspect of the oblique fissure (**Fig. 3**). On the left side, the upper half to two-thirds of the upper lobe is excised following a line that is nearly parallel to the oblique fissure. On both sides, respecting the posterior aspect of the fissure avoids damaging or tethering the superior segment of the lower lobe. Either could indeed prevent the superior segment from fully expanding and filling the apex of the chest. Care is taken to create a straight and single staple line. The resected specimen is then placed in an Endobag (EndoCatch Gold; Medtronic, Minneapolis, MN) and exteriorized through the utility incision or the 12-mm port, which may have to be enlarged in the face of a large resection.

With experience, the authors moved away from placing 2 chest tubes postoperatively to only one 24 or 28F straight tube with multiple additional holes whenever possible. This tube is exteriorized through the lowest port site. At the end of the procedure, the lung is reinflated under direct vision. Following this, the authors apply the lowest amount of suction possible that would keep the lung up, usually starting at -10 cm H_2O in the immediate postoperative period and rapidly moving to water seal. Indeed, minimal, if any, chest tube suction

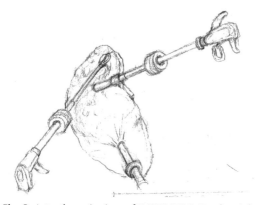

Fig. 3. Intrathoracic view of LVATS LVRS. On the right side, the staple line is started straight across the middle lobe beginning medially above the hilum. (*Courtesy of* Linda Capello, Sag Harbor, New York, USA.)

appears to decrease the severity and duration of postoperative air leaks.[10] Using the $Paco_2$-lowering strategy mentioned above, all the authors' patients are currently extubated in the operating room and then transferred awake to the ICU.

The Subxiphoid Video-Assisted Bilateral Thoracic Surgery Approach

Subxiphoid incisions have been used for decades by cardiothoracic surgeons to create pericardial windows. Reports dating back the late 1990s also demonstrated this approach was suitable to access the anterior mediastinum, especially for thymic resections.[18,19] As thoracic surgeons became more comfortable with the lateral uniportal approach for lung resections, the subxiphoid uniportal incision became more popular for thymic resections as well and proved suitable for pneumothorax surgery and lung resections, including segmentectomy and lobectomy.[20] It was therefore a quite natural evolution of the lateral uniportal VATS technique to move the incision subxiphoid for LVRS as well.[21,22] This midline incision is indeed ideally located to provide a minimal invasive bilateral pleural access. Since early 2019, the authors have adopted the subxiphoid video-assisted bilateral thoracic surgery (SVATS) access for all LVRS procedure at Columbia.

Technically, the authors perform a 2- to 3-cm incision on the midline below the xiphoid process. The subcutaneous fat is dissected, and the rectus muscles are spared by opening the linea alba. The substernal plane is then developed bluntly to create a working space, and the pleura is entered on the right side first. The authors do minimal substernal mobilization to avoid increasing postoperative pain. When the lung is fully freed, and in the absence incidental finding precluding to proceed with the procedure, the authors then place a 5-mm port laterally (**Fig. 4**). In the authors' early subxiphoid experience, they placed that port in the eighth or ninth intercostal space on the anterior axillary line, but they more recently moved the incision caudally to place the port totally subcostal. Subcostal port placement is then best achieved using 1 finger inside the chest to depress the diaphragm and place the port safely above the finger. The port should be placed at least 2 cm below the costal arch to avoid costal arch trauma, which can be painful, and should be aimed laterally during initial placement to avoid cardiac injury. The combination of this port with a 30-degree angled camera allows wide view and easy manipulation of the lung. LVRS can be thereafter carried out by inserting the lung retractor together with the stapler via the subxiphoid incision. The resection achieved through the subxiphoid incision is exactly the same as depicted using LVATS. At the end of the procedure, a single 24F or 28F straight chest tube is oriented apically in the pleural cavity and exteriorized through the subcostal port site (**Fig. 5**).

The left side is carried out similarly to the right. The major difference relates to the heart position that mandates a more lateral subcostal port placement and more careful port insertion to avoid any cardiac injury. Because of the heart position, the left side is technically somewhat more challenging than the right, and instruments must be entered cautiously. Heart compression during the procedure may generate some arrhythmias or hemodynamic instability. It is the authors' practice to operate on the easier right side first, as it further decreases compression to perform the left side in a more comfortable physiology.

The combination of subxiphoid midline incision and subcostal port placement allows fully extrathoracic access to further reduce the patient's pain. Similar to reports showing decreased pain with SVATS compared with LVATS,[23] the authors' experience reveals an average 2.3-fold decrease in patient's pain scores during the first 3 postoperative days when using the subxiphoid approach (Mark E. Ginsburg, MD, unpublished data). Such significant decrease in pain improved early mobilization and allowed the authors to move away from epidural requirements.

COMPLICATIONS OF LUNG VOLUME REDUCTION SURGERY

As the principal surgical complication, air leaks develop in most LVRS patients and are prolonged in half, which inevitably leads to a more complicated and longer hospital course. Their prevalence and duration are associated with certain patient characteristics, such as the use of inhaled steroids, worse pulmonary function, and distribution of disease (less common and shorter in lower lobe disease), and are more common and longer when extensive pleural adhesions are present. In contrast, surgical technique, such as choice of staple line buttressing material, use of pleural tents, or pleurodesis, does not seem to significantly prevent air leaks.[17] Some recent internal unpublished data also suggest that multiple resection lines, rather than the resected volume itself, are an independent risk factor for prolonged air leaks (Mark E. Ginsburg, MD, unpublished data). As depicted above, the most linear and therefore shortest staple line represents the ideal LVRS plan. Regarding space management, the authors do not perform pleural tents and no longer divide the pulmonary ligament. Infections are the second major complication following LVRS. Pneumonia is the most serious of these and is avoided by aggressive management of secretions and early mobilization. Although low-grade pleural contamination may help to promote pleural fusion, empyema is rare but may be severe.

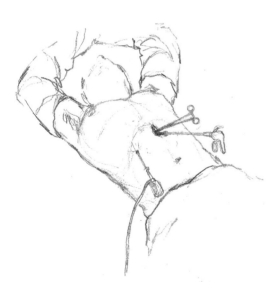

Fig. 4. Subxiphoid incision and lateral subcostal port placement for SVATS LVRS. A 2- to 3-cm midline subxiphoid access allows bilateral resections. A lateral 5-mm port is placed subcostal on each anterior axillary line to allow full extrathoracic approach. (*Courtesy of* Linda Capello, Sag Harbor, New York, USA.)

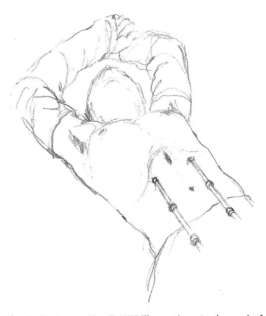

Fig. 5. Postoperative SVATS illustration. At the end of the procedure, a single 24F or 28F straight chest tube is oriented apically in the pleural cavity and exteriorized through the subcostal port site. (*Courtesy of* Linda Capello, Sag Harbor, New York, USA.)

SUMMARY

As a palliative treatment option, LVRS can be offered to a selected subset of COPD patients. Careful adherence to established inclusion and exclusion criteria is critical to achieve good outcomes. The evolution of surgical techniques toward minimally invasive VATS approaches has improved patient outcomes.[4] In addition, the authors have moved toward less aggressive surgical resections, and better match for the size of the hemithorax, and this has contributed to a short-term reduction in morbidity as well as to continued improvements in overall cardiopulmonary function. Recently, the fully extrathoracic access combining a midline subxiphoid incision with subcostal port placement allowed the authors to further decrease postoperative pain and favor early postoperative mobilization. With these techniques, the authors' patients experience improved pulmonary function tests, effort capacity, and dyspnea scores out to 5 years post-LVRS. Outcome at 1 year showed 99% survival; 5-year survival is 78%, and the authors' median survival is 9 years.

CLINICS CARE POINTS

- Fenestrate bullous areas to operate on a deflated lung and minimize manipulation of the fragile diseased lung to reduce air leaks.

- Avoid excessive volume reductions to minimize postoperative spaces.

- Before extubation, the permissive hypercapnia must be recognized and fully reversed to avoid and exacerbate the drowsiness associated with higher $Paco_2$ after extubation.

- Patients are best monitored in the intensive care unit for the first 24 to 48 postoperative hours.

- Chest tubes are connected to low suction until transition to water seal.

- Early aggressive incentive spirometry, physiotherapy, and mobilization are recommended.

- Early tracheostomy should be performed in patients who require reintubation.

REFERENCES

1. Brantigan OC, Mueller E, Kress MB. A surgical approach to pulmonary emphysema. Am Rev Respir Dis 1959;80(1, Part 2):194–206.
2. Fishman A, Martinez F, Naunheim K, et al. A randomized trial comparing lung-volume-reduction surgery with medical therapy for severe emphysema. N Engl J Med 2003;348(21):2059–73.
3. Licker M, Schweizer A, Ellenberger C, et al. Perioperative medical management of patients with COPD. Int J Chron Obstruct Pulmon Dis 2007;2(4):493–515.
4. Seadler B, Thuppal S, Rizvi N, et al. Clinical and quality of life outcomes after lung volume reduction surgery. Ann Thorac Surg 2019;108(3):866–72.
5. DeCamp MM Jr, McKenna RJ Jr, Deschamps CC, et al. Lung volume reduction surgery: technique, operative mortality, and morbidity. Proc Am Thorac Soc 2008;5(4):442–6.
6. Ginsburg ME, Thomashow BM, Bulman WA, et al. The safety, efficacy, and durability of lung-volume reduction surgery: a 10-year experience. J Thorac Cardiovasc Surg 2016;151(3):717–724 e711.
7. Donahue JM, Cassivi SD. Lung volume reduction surgery for patients with alpha-1 antitrypsin deficiency emphysema. Thorac Surg Clin 2009;19(2):201–8.
8. Perikleous P, Sharkey A, Oey I, et al. Long-term survival and symptomatic relief in lower lobe lung volume reduction surgery. Eur J Cardiothorac Surg 2017;52(5):982–8.
9. Brantigan OC, Mueller E. Surgical treatment of pulmonary emphysema. Am Surg 1957;23(9):789–804.
10. Cooper JD, Trulock EP, Triantafillou AN, et al. Bilateral pneumectomy (volume reduction) for chronic obstructive pulmonary disease. J Thorac Cardiovasc Surg 1995;109(1):106–16 [discussion 116–09].
11. Friscia ME, Zhu J, Kolff JW, et al. Cytokine response is lower after lung volume reduction through bilateral thoracoscopy versus sternotomy. Ann Thorac Surg 2007;83(1):252–6.
12. McKenna RJ Jr, Benditt JO, DeCamp M, et al. Safety and efficacy of median sternotomy versus video-assisted thoracic surgery for lung volume reduction surgery. J Thorac Cardiovasc Surg 2004;127(5):1350–60.
13. McKenna RJ Jr, Brenner M, Fischel RJ, et al. Should lung volume reduction for emphysema be unilateral or bilateral? J Thorac Cardiovasc Surg 1996;112(5):1331–8 [discussion 1338–9].
14. Rationale and design of the National Emphysema Treatment Trial: a prospective randomized trial of lung volume reduction surgery. The National Emphysema Treatment Trial Research Group. Chest 1999;116(6):1750–61.
15. Stammberger U, Klepetko W, Stamatis G, et al. Buttressing the staple line in lung volume reduction surgery: a randomized three-center study. Ann Thorac Surg 2000;70(6):1820–5.
16. Hazelrigg SR, Boley TM, Naunheim KS, et al. Effect of bovine pericardial strips on air leak after stapled pulmonary resection. Ann Thorac Surg 1997;63(6):1573–5.
17. DeCamp MM, Blackstone EH, Naunheim KS, et al. Patient and surgical factors influencing air leak after

lung volume reduction surgery: lessons learned from the National Emphysema Treatment Trial. Ann Thorac Surg 2006;82(1):197–206 [discussion 206–197].

18. Abu-Akar F, Gonzalez-Rivas D, Yang C, et al. Subxiphoid uniportal VATS for thymic and combined mediastinal and pulmonary resections - a two-year experience. Semin Thorac Cardiovasc Surg 2019; 31(3):614–9.

19. Akamine S, Takahashi T, Oka T, et al. Thymic cystectomy through subxyphoid by video-assisted thoracic surgery. Ann Thorac Surg 1999;68(6):2339–41.

20. Ali J, Haiyang F, Aresu G, et al. Uniportal subxiphoid video-assisted thoracoscopic anatomical segmentectomy:

technique and results. Ann Thorac Surg 2018;106(5): 1519–24.

21. Akar FA. Subxiphoid uniportal approach is it just a trend or the future of VATS. MOJ Surg 2017;4(4): 70–1.

22. Nashaat A, Aresu G, Peryt A, et al. Subxiphoid uniportal video-assisted thoracoscopic lung volume reduction surgery. Interact Cardiovasc Thorac Surg 2019;28(3):485–6.

23. Li L, Tian H, Yue W, et al. Subxiphoid vs intercostal single-incision video-assisted thoracoscopic surgery for spontaneous pneumothorax: a randomised controlled trial. Int J Surg 2016;30:99–103.

Alpha₁-antitrypsin Disease, Treatment and Role for Lung Volume Reduction Surgery

Nathalie Foray, DO, MS*, Taylor Stone, MD, Peter White, MD

KEYWORDS

- Alpha₁-antitrypsin deficiency • Chronic obstructive pulmonary disease
- Lung volume reduction surgery • AATD-related pulmonary emphysema
- Endobronchial lung volume reduction

KEY POINTS

- There are 5 published series of severe alpha₁-antitrypsin disease (AATD) patients who underwent lung volume reduction surgery (LVRS) and 3 published series of severe AATD patients who underwent endoscopic lung volume reduction (ELVR).
- The improvement in forced expiratory volume in the first second of expiration (FEV_1) was on average not sustained, such that by 12 months to 24 months only 2 LRVS and 1 ELVR series reported that the FEV_1 remained higher than the baseline value.
- In the 4 series with data at 3 months to 8 months postprocedure, 4 found a statistically significant decrease in dyspnea scores and there was a statistically significant decrease in dyspnea scores in 3 of 6 studies by 12 months to 24 months postprocedure.

INTRODUCTION TO CHRONIC OBSTRUCTIVE PULMONARY DISEASE
Chronic Obstructive Pulmonary Disease/Emphysema: Pathology and Physiology

Chronic obstructive pulmonary disease (COPD) is described as airflow obstruction that not always is reversible and usually is subcategorized into 2 groups: chronic bronchitis and emphysema.[1,2] In 2015, the Global Burden of Disease study estimated global prevalence of COPD at approximately 174 million cases, which likely represents an undercount.[3] The same year, COPD ranked as third leading cause of death, with 3.2 million people dying from the disease.[3]

Chronic bronchitis and emphysema are differentiated based on anatomy. Chronic bronchitis is defined by permanent obstruction of the airways, with a forced expiratory volume in the first second of expiration (FEV_1) to forced vital capacity (FVC) ratio of less than 70%.[1] Emphysema is an anatomic description of the destruction of alveolar walls beyond the terminal bronchioles.[1] Centrilobular emphysema is associated with cigarette smoking, whereas panacinar (panlobular) emphysema commonly is found in individuals with alpha₁-antitrypsin disease (AATD). Both patterns can be seen in the same patient.[1]

The main cause of COPD is smoking.[1–3] Smoke inhalation causes inflammatory cells to infiltrate the bronchiole mucosa, submucosa, and glandular tissue, leading to increased mucus, hyperplasia of epithelial cells, bronchial wall thickening, and

Conflicts of Interest: None of the authors that contributed to this article have any conflicts of interest, not limited to commercial, financial, or any funding sources.
Department of Internal Medicine, Division of Pulmonary and Critical Care Medicine, Southern Illinois University School of Medicine, 801 North Rutledge Street, Room 1269, Springfield, IL 62702, USA
* Corresponding author.
E-mail address: nforay@siumed.edu

impairment of tissue repair.[2] These lead to airway remodeling and emphysema with loss of elastic recoil, which subsequently cause a decrease in FEV_1, enhance gas trapping, and lead to hyperinflation and dyspnea.[2,3]

Treatment

Smoking cessation

Smoking cessation is imperative to reduce the accelerated decline of lung function over time as well as the associated exacerbations and comorbidities.[3] If initiated early, smoking cessation can decrease the incidence of respiratory morbidity.[4] The Lung Health Study in 1994 found that in individuals with mild or moderate COPD (FEV_1 >50%), intensive smoking cessation programs were associated with improvements in lung function at 5 years.[4] Various modalities, both pharmacologic and nonpharmacologic, are available to help with smoking cessation.[3]

Bronchodilators

Maintenance pharmacotherapy is used in those with stable COPD to improve symptoms and quality-of-life, decrease exacerbations and improve exercise tolerance.[3] Inhaled long-acting $β_2$-agonists (LABAs), long-acting antimuscarinic antagonists (LAMAs), and inhaled corticosteroids (ICSs) are used individually or in combination for maintenance therapy. Inhaled LABA and ICSs have been known to decrease exacerbations.[5] The addition of LAMA to LABA/ICS therapy is associated with fewer exacerbations than LABA/ICSs alone.[3]

Anti-inflammatory drugs

Patients whose COPD remains poorly controlled despite maximal inhaler regimens may require oral pharmacotherapy. Roflumilast is a phosphodiesterase-4 inhibitor that may reduce airway inflammation and bronchoconstriction.[3,6] Roflumilast decreases exacerbations requiring corticosteroid treatment but has not been shown to improve life expectancy or quality of life.[6] Macrolide antibiotics have been studied for continuous or intermittent use in COPD and may decrease exacerbations and hospitalizations as well as improve quality of life.[3]

Exacerbations, antibiotics, and systemic steroids

Exacerbations of COPD usually involve increased sputum, cough, and dyspnea.[2,3] Mild exacerbations can be treated with bronchodilators, moderate exacerbations require antibiotics and often systemic steroids, and severe exacerbations often require hospitalization.[2] Exacerbations are associated with worsening disease progression, decreased quality of life, and increased risk of mortality.[2] The most frequent cause for COPD exacerbations is a viral or bacterial infection.[2] In those with severe exacerbations requiring hospital admission, 78% of the cases were identified as being cause by infection.[2]

Current guidelines recommend, in the absence of contraindications, that oral corticosteroids should be used with other therapies in all patients hospitalized with acute exacerbations.[7] The role of systemic steroids in the outpatient setting is unclear.[7] A 5-day duration of corticosteroids is noninferior to a 14-day course.[7,8]

Supplemental oxygen and non-invasive ventilation

In 1980, the Nocturnal Oxygen Therapy Trial Group compared continuous oxygen therapy (24 h/d) with 12-hour nocturnal oxygen therapy in individuals with hypoxemic COPD.[9] At 2-year follow-up, continuous oxygen therapy was found associated with lower mortality compared with the nocturnal oxygen group.[9,10] In 1981, the UK Medical Research Council (MRC) trial randomly allocated patients with COPD and severe hypoxemia to receive oxygen (at least 15 h/d) or no oxygen.[10,11] The 5-year difference in mortality was 21% in favor of those using supplemental oxygen. These 2 trials established long-term oxygen therapy as the standard of care. For years it was assumed that oxygen for nocturnal and exercise-induced hypoxemia also was beneficial.[10] In 2018, it was shown that the use of supplemental oxygen in patients with exercise-induced hypoxemia (but normal resting oxygen levels) improved exercise capacity but had no impact on survival or quality of life.[12] Similarly, the role of supplemental nocturnal oxygen for patients with isolated nocturnal hypoxemia recently has been called into question.[13] Despite this, the use of supplemental oxygen for exercise-induced hypoxemia and isolated nocturnal hypoxemia remains widespread.

Pulmonary rehabilitation

Pulmonary rehabilitation (PR) improves exercise tolerance in those patients with COPD. PR is recommended for patients with COPD who also have a modified (mMRC) dyspnea scale score of greater than or equal to 2.[14] In these individuals, PR increased exercise capacity and quality of life and decreased dyspnea and BODE index.[15,16] PR has been described as a cost-effective way to reduce hospital admissions and mortality in patients who have had severe exacerbations. Despite this, PR remains underutilized worldwide.[3]

Prognosis and Mortality Risk

Mortality from COPD is higher for men, those with severe disease, and those greater than 45 years of age.[1] Prognosis after hospitalization is poor.[3] The mortality rate during hospitalization for a COPD exacerbation ranges from 2.5% to 10%.[1] This increases with time post-hospitalization, with a mortality rate of 16% to 19% at 3 months post-hospitalization, 23% to 43% at 1 year post-hospitalization, and 55% to 60% at 5 years.[1] Comorbidities also are a major cause of hospitalization and death in COPD patients.[17] The only factors that have been shown to yield a decrease in mortality have been smoking cessation and long-term oxygen therapy in those with chronic respiratory failure from COPD.[1]

ALPHA₁-ANTITRYPSIN DISEASE
History

René Laennec described the clinical features, pathology, diagnosis, and treatment of emphysema in his 1826 *Treatise on Mediate Auscultation and Diseases of the Chest*.[18,19] His views on emphysema heavily influenced pulmonary physicians for the next 135 years. By the 1960s, researchers were beginning to examine the molecular basis for emphysema, focusing on the destruction of the connective tissue scaffolding of emphysematous lungs.[18] In 1964, Laurell and Eriksson[20] published their seminal work on AATD. They analyzed 1500 samples of serum via paper electrophoresis and discovered that 5 samples lacked a band, which they correctly identified as AATD (**Fig. 1**). Three of the 5 cases were symptomatic, having developed pulmonary emphysema at a young age. Two of the patients lacked obvious pulmonary disease but 1 of these had a familial history

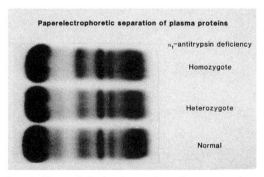

Fig. 1. The original electrophoretic preparations. (*From* Sandhaus RA, Turino G, Brantly ML, et al. Clinical practice guidelines: The diagnosis and management of alpha-1 antitrypsin deficiency in the adult. J COPD Found. 2016;3(3):668–82; with permission. Taylor & Francis Ltd, http://www.tandfonline.com.)

of pulmonary emphysema. Further work by Eriksson[21] demonstrated the heterogeneous nature of disease in patients with AATD, with some experiencing severe early-onset obstructive lung disease and others manifesting no clinical symptoms. Laurell and Eriksson's[20] discovery of the role of AATD in the pathogenesis of panacinar emphysema led to the so-called proteolytic theory of emphysema, in which proteases are released by pulmonary neutrophils and macrophages, leading to excessive proteolytic activity in the lungs and subsequent tissue destruction.[18] This theory gained support when it was demonstrated in 1964 that emphysema could be induced in rat lungs by the intratracheal instillation of papain into rat lungs.[22]

Pathophysiology of Alpha₁-antitrypsin Disease

A more detailed understanding of the genetics and biochemistry of AATD has been elucidated since Laurell and Eriksson's initial findings in 1963. AATD is a member of the serine protease inhibitor (SERPIN) superfamily.[23] Most people possess 2 copies of the wild-type M-allele of the SERPINA1 gene, which encodes the AATD protein. People with the Pi*MM genotype, where Pi stands for protease inhibitor, have normal serum levels of functional AATD. AATD primarily is synthesized within hepatocytes, although it also is produced within intestinal cells, pulmonary alveolar cells, white blood cells, and the cornea. It is synthesized within the endoplasmic reticulum before being trafficked via the Golgi apparatus and ultimately secreted into the plasma. AATD most commonly is the result of deficiency alleles, in which a mutant AATD protein is synthesized, with the majority being destroyed within the endoplasmic reticulum prior to secretion (70%) and smaller proportions being secreted (15%) or going on to form polymers (15%), which themselves are degraded via autophagy or secreted into the plasma. The Z (Glu342Lys) allele is 1 such deficiency allele and is responsible for 95% of severe AATD cases. The Z allele is found in 1 in 25 people with European ancestry and 1 in 2000 people with European ancestry are homozygotes for Z (Pi*ZZ), making AATD 1 of the most common inherited disorders among white persons (**Fig. 2**). Other deficiency alleles result in misfolded proteins, varying degrees of polymerization, intracellular degradation, abnormal posttranslational biosynthesis, and unstable protein structure. The S (Glu264Val) allele is even more common than the Z allele, with a carrier frequency of 1:4 people in the Iberian Peninsula, 1:5 people in southern Europe, and 1:30

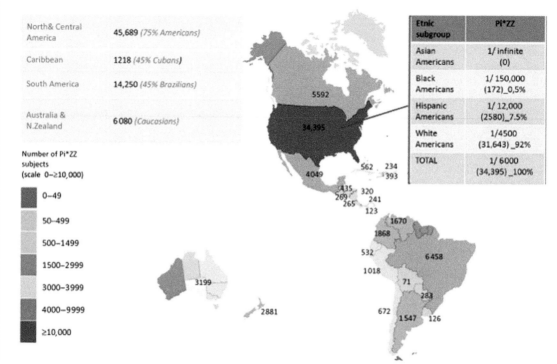

Etnic subgroup	Pi*ZZ
Asian Americans	1/ infinite (0)
Black Americans	1/ 150,000 (172)_0,5%
Hispanic Americans	1/ 12,000 (2580)_7.5%
White Americans	1/4500 (31,643)_92%
TOTAL	1/ 6000 (34,395)_100%

North& Central America 45,689 (75% Americans)

Caribbean 1218 (45% Cubans)

South America 14,250 (45% Brazilians)

Australia & N.Zealand 6080 (Caucasians)

Number of Pi*ZZ subjects (scale 0–≥10,000)

0–49

50–499

500–1499

1500–2999

3000–3999

4000–9999

≥10,000

Fig. 2. Role of AATD in human health and disease. Pi*ZZ numbers and distribution. (*From* de Serres F, Blanco I. Role of alpha-1 antitrypsin in human health and disease. J Intern Med. 2014;276: 311–35; with permission.)

people in the United States. Individuals with Pi*SS, Pi*MZ, and Pi*SZ generally have AATD levels reduced to 40% to 60% of normal, compared with 15% of normal for Pi*ZZ individuals. They may be at increased risk of emphysema but it is not as severe as in Pi*ZZ homozygotes. In addition to the deficiency alleles, there are several null (Pi*QO) alleles, in which there is either no detectable AATD mRNA, or a truncated, nonfunctional protein is synthesized but not secreted.

In the lungs, AATD inhibits neutrophil elastase, a proteolytic enzyme thought to be the key enzyme involved in the pathologic degradation of pulmonary elastin.[23] Instillation of neutrophil elastase in model animals leads to airspace enlargement, and neutrophil elastase knockout mice are protected from smoking-induced emphysema.[18] AATD has been shown to inhibit neutrophil elastase in vivo and prevent lung digestion by leukoproteases in vitro. AATD has a 1000-fold more rapid rate of association with neutrophil elastase than with trypsin, further supporting neutrophil elastase inhibition as its most important function. Among AATD patients, it is thought that insufficient quantities of slower-acting mutant AATD reach the lungs, leading to unchecked activity of neutrophil elastase and resultant tissue destruction (**Fig. 3**).[23] Polymerized Z AATD has a proinflammatory effect in the lungs, attracting neutrophils and

increasing proteolytic activity, ultimately leading to structural damage and increased susceptibility to infection. Oxidation also plays an important role in inactivation of AATD. A methionine residue at the active site of AATD may be oxidized in the presence of chemical oxidants, myeloperoxidase, or cigarette smoke.[18] AATD methionine oxidation

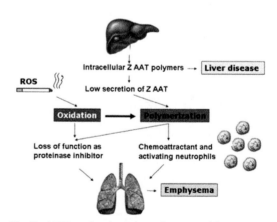

Fig. 3. AATD pathophysiology. (Reprinted from Respiratory Medicine, Vol 105/Issue 8, Janciauskiene SM, Bals R, Koczulla R, Vogelmeier C, Köhnlein T, Welte T, The discovery of α1-antitrypsin and its role in health and disease, 1129-1139, copyright 2011, with permission from Elsevier.)

results in a loss of biologic activity. This discovery led to the development of the oxidation hypothesis, which seeks to explain smoker's emphysema in patients with normal plasma levels of AATD as being due to increased inactivation of AATD by oxidative stress from cigarette smoke.

Systemic Disease in Alpha₁-antitrypsin Disease

Patients with AATD also are susceptible to liver disease, although the mechanism differs from the loss-of-function seen in AATD emphysema.[23] Misfolded Z AATD polymerizes within hepatocytes, resulting in proteotoxic stress and gain-of-function liver disease. Clinically significant liver fibrosis is seen in 20% to 35% of Pi*ZZ AATD patients. In addition to the more common emphysema and liver disease, several systemic disorders also have been associated with AATD in persons with the Pi*ZZ genotype. Severe adult asthma, necrotizing panniculitis, antineutrophil cytoplasmic vasculitis (ANCA)-associated vasculitis, chronic kidney disease, diabetes, and metabolic alterations all are overrepresented in patients with the Pi*ZZ allele.[23,24]

Lung Disease in Alpha₁-antitrypsin Disease

AATD-related pulmonary emphysema is seen most commonly in Pi*ZZ genotypes (95% of cases).[24] Penetrance is approximately 60% in Pi*ZZ individuals. AATD-related pulmonary emphysema in Pi*ZZ individuals is thought to be responsible for approximately 1% to 2% of all COPD cases.[25] Symptoms largely are indistinguishable from the garden variety smoker's emphysema seen in individuals with normal serum AATD levels, making underdiagnosis and diagnostic delays common.[23] Pulmonary symptoms, such as cough, dyspnea, and sputum production, may be seen by the fourth to fifth decades of life.[25] Bronchial hyperreactivity may be seen in up to 20% of symptomatic patients, and bronchodilator response is a risk factor for FEV₁ decline. Early-onset obstructive lung disease with imaging findings of lower lobe–predominant panacinar emphysema in a patient with moderate smoking history is the classic clinical description of AATD-associated lung disease (**Fig. 4**).[23] Recent studies have shown that approximately two-thirds of AATD subjects have a predominantly basal pattern whereas approximately one-third have greater involvement in the apical regions.[26] Presumably, the basilar predilection among AATD patients is due to the effects of gravity on pulmonary perfusion and the migration of hematogenous inflammatory cells, although the exact mechanism

remains unknown.[26] Likewise, approximately three-quarters of AATD-related emphysema subjects were noted to have panacinar emphysema, whereas approximately one-third were noted to have centrilobular emphysema.[27] Approximately 27% of AATD-associated emphysema patients have bronchiectasis on CT.[27]

Due to the lack of specific demographic and clinical characteristics, it is recommended that all patients with COPD should be tested for AATD, regardless of smoking history.[28] Testing also is recommended in patients with unexplained chronic liver disease, severe adult asthma, unexplained bronchiectasis, ANCA and systemic vasculitis, and relapsing panniculitis.[24] Severe AATD deficiency is defined as serum levels less than 35% of the mean expected value (80 mg/dL, or 11 μmol/L measured by radial immunodiffusion).[24]

Treatment of Alpha₁-antitrypsin Disease

Response to bronchodilators, ICSs, PR, supplemental oxygen therapy, and immunizations is not significantly different than in AATD-replete COPD patients.[28] As such, treatment algorithms are not significantly different for AATD-associated emphysema compared with AATD-replete COPD. Every effort should be made to prevent exposure to tobacco or to facilitate cessation in those who smoke given increased rates of decline in lung function compared with those with AATD-replete COPD. Intravenous augmentation therapy with purified preparations of pooled donor-derived human AATD is recommended for patients with an FEV₁ in the range of 30% to 65% of predicted. Intravenous augmentation has been shown to decrease elastin degradation and rates of loss of CT lung density compared with placebo in individuals with AATD-associated emphysema. The use of intravenous augmentation in patients with FEV₁ less than 30% is debated.[28,29] Recent guidelines recommend the use of augmentation therapy in this population.[28] Current smokers have not been shown to benefit from intravenous augmentation therapy and should not be offered treatment until they achieve smoking cessation. Intravenous augmentation therapy also is not recommended for Pi*MZ patients or other heterozygote genotypes with a normal M gene. Current guidelines recommend against LVRS in AATD patients on the basis of prior studies showing short-lived benefits compared with AATD-replete COPD patients and basilar predominance of emphysema in AATD, making LRVS more technically challenging.[28] The National Emphysema Treatment Trial (NETT) also found higher mortality among AATD patients treated with LVRS compared with those treated

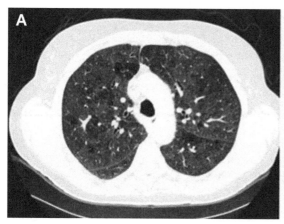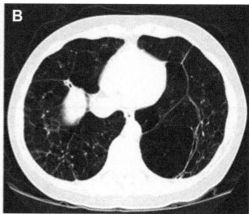

Fig. 4. Computed tomography in AATD. (*A*) Emphysematous changes at the level of the aortic arch. (*B*) emphysematous changes above the diaphragm in the lower lung zones. (Reprinted from Thoracic Surgery Clinics, Vol 19/Edition 2, Donahue JM, Cassivi SD, Lung volume reduction surgery for patients with alpha-1 antitrypsin deficiency emphysema, 201-8, copyright 2009, with permission from Elsevier.)

with medical management alone.[30] There currently is no specific treatment of AATD-associated liver disease.[28]

LUNG VOLUME REDUCTION SURGERY
History

Lung volume reduction surgery (LVRS) can trace it roots to the 1950s in Baltimore, Maryland. Dr Otto Brantigan (**Fig. 5**) and colleagues[31] described the surgical techniques and respiratory

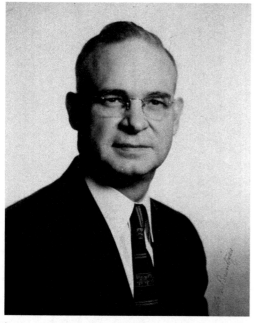

Fig. 5. Dr Otto Brantigan. (*Courtesy of* U.S. National Library of Medicine via University of Maryland School of Medicine, Baltimore, Maryland.)

pathophysiology that form the basis for modern day LVRS surgery. Brantigan reasoned that in patients with "idiopathic hypertrophic obstructive pulmonary emphysema," the removal of the periphery of the upper lobes would reduce lung hyperinflation, restore lung "elasticity" and the circumferential pull that tethers open the bronchioles (**Fig. 6**), improve diaphragmatic mechanics and possibly improve cardiac function. Brantigan and colleagues performed staged bilateral thoracotomies utilizing a clamp and suture technique to remove the periphery of the upper lobes. Brantigan and colleagues[31] reported a series of 31 patients who underwent LVRS. There were 6 postoperative deaths (19%) but no deaths after the second surgery. They reported all but 1 patient who survived the first surgery "benefited." Pulmonary function tests (PFTs) results were not reported but they noted that some patients had no improvement in measure pulmonary function after surgery but breath sounds and exercise capacity was "greatly improved." The operation subsequently was abandoned due to high operative mortality and inconsistent results.[32]

In the 1990s, LVRS was resurrected by Joel Cooper and colleagues.[33] They performed bilateral LVRS via a median sternotomy and removed 20% to 30% of the upper lobes using an endostapler with reinforced bovine pericardium. Their case series showed benefit both in terms of PFT values and exercise capacity. Cooper and colleagues reported results from 150 patients who had undergone bilateral LVRS via median sternotomy. Six months after surgery, the average improvement in PFT values were impressive: 51% increase in FEV_1, 14% decrease in total lung capacity (TLC), and 28% decrease in residual volume (RV). The

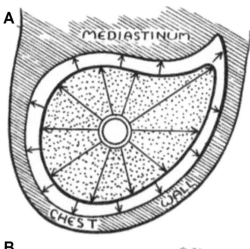

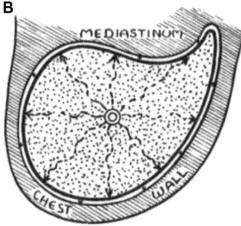

Fig. 6. Tethering of the bronchiole. (*A*) Schematic of an elastic lung showing bronchioles held open. (*B*) illustration of an emphysematous lung exceeding pleural space capacity and thus bronchioles are not held open. (Reprinted with permission of the American Thoracic Society. Copyright © 2020 American Thoracic Society. All rights reserved. Otto C Brantigan, Eugene Mueller, and Milton B. Kress, 1958, A Surgical Approach to Pulmonary Emphysema/American Review of Respiratory Disease*, Volume 80 (1P2), 194-206. The American Review of Respiratory Disease* is an official journal of the American Thoracic Society.)

average improvement in 6-minute walk distance (6MWD) after 6 months was 19%, and the percent of patients requiring supplemental oxygen with exercise went from 95% prior to surgery to 43% 6 months after surgery. Likewise, 6 months after LVRS, 98% of patients rated their health as somewhat or much better on the 36-Item Short Form Health Survey questionnaire (SF-36). The perioperative mortality rate was 4%.

Cooper and colleagues' results garnered substantial enthusiasm and set off a resurgence of interest in LVRS. LVRS was widely adopted with numerous technical modifications. This fervor for LVRS waned in response concerns for patient safety and surging health care costs.[34,35] The data supporting LVRS were based on nonrandomized case series with short-term follow-up, inconsistent selection criteria, and no agreement on what defined patient benefit.[34,35]

The National Emphysema Treatment Trial

The NETT started enrolling patients in January of 1998. Prior to completing the study, they reported that patients with an FEV₁ less than 20% of predicted and either homogeneous emphysema or a diffusing capacity for carbon monoxide (DLCO); less than 20% of predicted had high 30-day postoperative mortality (16% in the LVRS group vs 0 for the medical group) and they were unlikely to have functional improvement.[30] The NETT was completed in July 2002. It enrolled 1218 patients (608 LVRS group and 610 medical treatment group) with advanced emphysema (FEV₁ <45% predicted, TLC >100% predicted, and RV >150% predicted) from 17 US medical centers.[30] The NETT compared LVRS plus PR to optimal medical therapy plus PR. The primary endpoints were mortality and maximum exercise capacity at 24 months. Overall, LVRS was found to improve exercise capacity but have no effect on mortality (0.11 deaths per person-year in both groups). Exercise capacity at 24 months improved by greater than 10 W in 15% of the LVRS group versus 3% of patients in the optimal medical therapy group. Post hoc analysis identified 4 groups based on distribution of emphysema (upper lobe predominant versus non–upper lobe predominant) and exercise capacity (high exercise capacity low exercise capacity). In patients with predominantly upper lobe emphysema and low baseline exercise capacity, LVRS yielded a survival advantage over the medical therapy group (50% reduction in mortality). In the predominantly non–upper lobe emphysema and high baseline exercise capacity group, mortality in the LVRS group was twice as high as the medical therapy group, and there was no improvement in exercise capacity. In the predominantly upper lobe emphysema and high baseline exercise capacity group and the predominantly non–upper lobe emphysema and low baseline exercise capacity group, there was negligible improvement in exercise capacity but no improvement in survival. A subsequent meta-analysis of LVRS also found that patients with advanced heterogeneous emphysema and low exercise tolerance based on 6MWD experienced better functional outcomes from LVRS than from medical therapy.[36]

Surgical Approaches

Varying surgical techniques are used for LVRS but most commonly median sternotomy, thoracotomy, or bilateral video-assisted thoracoscopic surgery (VATS) are employed.[37] In the NETT data set, there was no significant difference in mortality, morbidity, or functional improvement between thoracotomy and median sternotomy.[30] The VATS approach has been reported to decrease hospital cost and length of stay. The LVRS procedure, regardless of the initial incision, requires the resection of 20% to 30% of each lung using an endostapler with a continuous staple line reinforced with bovine pericardial strips to mitigate the development of air leaks (**Fig. 7**). Emphysematous lung is left behind to avoid creating mismatch between the size of the lung and volume of thoracic cavity. In general, patients are extubated within 1 hour of completing the procedure. Chest tubes are placed to water seal in attempt to minimize transpulmonary pressure and reduce air leaks. Patients commonly require aggressive postoperative bronchial hygiene. The most common postoperative complications are prolonged air leaks and pneumonia.[30,33]

Endobronchial valves are discussed elsewhere in this issue. In general, 3 to 5 one-way valves are placed in the bronchi of the most severely affected lobes to decompress the over inflated emphysematous lung and direct the air to less affected regions of the lung (**Fig. 8**). In individuals

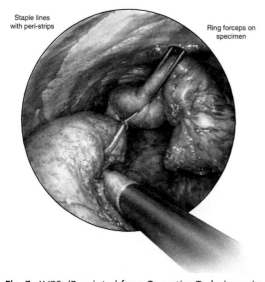

Fig. 7. LVRS. (Reprinted from Operative Techniques in Thoracic and Cardiovascular Surgery, Vol 12/Issue 2, McKenna, RJ. Thorascopic Lung Volume Reduction Surgery, 141-149, copyright 2007, with permission from Elsevier.)

with severe AATD, the values typically are placed in the lower lobe bronchi. When endobronchial valves are successful, the patient experiences the physiologic benefits of LVRS without having to undergo major thoracic surgery.

Physiology of Lung Volume Reduction Surgery

The mechanisms that result in the physiologic improvement following LVRS are not precisely known.[38] Reducing the size mismatch between the hyperinflated, floppy emphysematous lungs and the overdistended chest cavity is believed to play a central role in the physiologic improvement following successful LVRS. Restoring the size mismatch between the lungs and chest wall should improve the elastic recoil of the lung and thereby help to tether open the small and medium-sized airways, which would prevent premature airway closure and improve expiratory airflow.[39,40] It also may reduce exercise-induced dynamic hyperinflation and thereby decrease exertional breathlessness.[39] Sciurba and colleagues[41] reported that improved lung elastic recoil after LVRS was associated with increased exercise capacity. Decreasing lung and chest wall hyperinflation would help to restore the curvature of the diaphragm and place it on a more advantageous part of its length tension curve.[42] The effect should be similar for the intercostal and scalene muscles. Overall, there would be improved synchrony between the diaphragm, the intercostal muscles, the scalene muscles, and the other inspiratory muscles, resulting in amelioration of the chronic fatigue seen in the respiratory muscles of individuals with severe emphysema.[42,43] Relieving lung hyperinflation also may benefit cardiac performance by allowing improved left ventricular filling decreased left ventricular end-diastolic pressure.[38] The physiologic benefit of endobronchial valves is believed to be similar to LVRS.

Lung Reduction Surgery in Alpha₁-antitrypsin Disease

There are 5 published series of severe AATD patients who underwent LVRS and 3 published series of severe AATD patients who underwent endoscopic lung volume reduction (ELVR).[44–51] **Table 1** compares baseline characteristics among the 8 published series. The studies ranged from n = 6 to n = 20, for a total of 107 patients; 76 patients underwent LVRS and 41 underwent ELVR via endobronchial valve. A majority of patients studied were men, ranging from 47% to 83% in the 5 studies that broke down participants by sex. The average age ranged between 48 years and

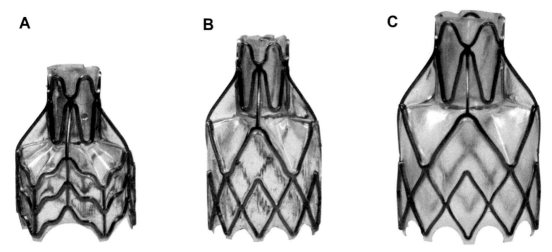

Fig. 8. Endobronchial valves. (A) EBV-TS-4.0-LP. (B) EBV-TS-4.0. (C) EBV-TS-5.5. (*Courtesy of* PulmonX, Redwood City, California; with permission.)

65 years. In the 4 series that reported the prevalence of prior cigarette smoking, 72% of patients were former cigarette smokers. All of the 64 patients with reported AATD levels had severe deficiency (<12 mmol/L or <65 mg/dL) and 96% (69/72) had the Pi*ZZ allele. Nearly three-quarters (70/95) of patients had the classic AATD distribution of lower lobe predominant emphysema in the 7 series that reported distribution.

Tables 2 and **3** list the inclusion and exclusion criteria, respectively, for 8 series. Age was listed as an inclusion criterion in 3 series (>60, ≤80 years, and ≥40 years) and as an exclusion criterion in 2 series (>75 years in both). These series included severe airflow obstruction, hyperinflation, air trapping, and severe exercise limitation as inclusion criteria, although the specific operational definitions varied. FEV_1 was listed in 5 series and varied between 35% and 45%; Cassina and colleagues[44] listed an absolute FEV_1 of less than 1.1 L as a cutoff. Hyperinflation, as measured by TLC, was listed in 5 series, and cutoffs varied from greater than 100% to greater than 130% of predicted. Air trapping, as measured by RV, was listed in 4 series and cutoff values varied from greater than 140% to greater than 200% of predicted. Severe dyspnea was used in 7 series and was defined by a validated score in all but 1 series. Poor quality of life was an inclusion criterion in 7 series but only Cassina and colleagues[44] used a validated scoring system (SF-36 questionnaire) to quantify the patients' quality of life.[44] All of the series used computed tomography scans to determine the presence of heterogeneous emphysema. Three of the series (1 LVRS series and 2 ELVR series) did not provide exclusion criteria. Active cigarette smoking was an explicit

exclusion criterion in 2 series. Only 1 series (Tutic and colleagues[46]) used PFT data: DLCO less than 20% was an exclusion criterion. Elevated resting room air $Paco_2$ is a marker of chronic respiratory failure and 2 series used an elevated $Paco_2$ as an exclusion criterion with cutoff values of greater than 48 mm Hg (>6.4 kPa) and greater than 55 mm Hg (>7.3 kPa). Four series excluded bronchiectasis and 3 series excluded pulmonary hypertension (mean pulmonary artery pressure >35 mm Hg [>4.7 kPa]). Two series listed heart failure with reduced ejection fraction (HFrEF) as an exclusion criterion, 1 series excluded malignancy with a left expectancy less than 2 years, and 2 series excluded patients on chronic steroids (>15 mg/d of prednisolone equivalent). Inclusion/exclusion criteria varied widely between these case series despite all of the patients having severe AATD and advanced emphysema.

Table 4 describes the characteristics of the operation performed. Among the 5 LVRS studies, 3 were bilateral, 1 was unilateral, and 1 included both unilateral and bilateral operations (the majority being bilateral). Two of the LVRS series were performed exclusively via VATS, 2 were performed exclusively via thoracotomy, and 1 was done via VATS or thoracotomy. All of the ELVR studies were performed by unilateral placement of endobronchial valves.

Table 5 lists the spirometry and plethysmography data at baseline and the best postprocedure results between 3 months and 8 months and between 12 months and 24 months. The initial average FEV_1 ranged between 18% and 30% of predicted, which is compatible with very severe airflow obstruction. Seven of the series reported

Table 1
Baseline characteristics

Series	N	Women (%)	Age (y), mean ±SD	Prior Cigarette Smoker (%)	Alpha$_1$-antitrypsin <12 µmol/L (%)	Pi*ZZ (%)	Augmentation Therapy (%)	Emphysema Distribution Lower Lobe Predominance
Cassina et al,[44] 1998	12	5 (42)	49 ± 10	5 (42)	12 (100)	12 (100)	12 (100)	ND
Gelb et al,[45] 1999	6	1 (17)	61 ± 9	4 (67)	6 (100)	6 (100)	5 (50)	6 (100)
Tutic et al,[46] 2004 50	21	10 (48)	56 ± 2	19 (90.5)	21 (100)	18 (86)	1 (5)	10 (48)
Dauriat et al,[47] 2006	17	ND	56 ± 9	ND	15 (ND in 2 patients)	15 (ND in 2 patients)	ND	17 (100)
Stoller et al,[48] 2007	10	2 (20)	65.8 (55.4–77.0)[a]	ND	10 (100)	ND	ND	3 (30)
Tuohy et al,[49] 2011	6	1 (17)	48	ND	6 (100)	6 (100)	ND	6 (67)
Hillerdal et al,[50] 2014	15	8 (53)	64	11 (73)	ND	15 (100)	0 (0)	13 (87)
Delage et al,[51] 2019	20	ND	ND	ND	ND	ND	ND	17 (85)

Abbreviation: ND, no data.
[a] Reported as median (quartiles).

Table 2
Inclusion criteria

Series	Age (y)	Severe Obstruction	Hyperinflation and Air Trapping	Severe Dyspnea	Impaired Quality of Life	Heterogeneous Emphysema on Lung Imaging	Matched V/Q Defects	Other
Cassina et al,[44] 1998	N/A	FEV$_1$ ≤1.1 L, TLC >120% of predicted	TLC >120% of predicted	MRC >2	Yes; SF-36	Yes	Yes	No bulla >5 cm
Gelb et al,[45] 1999	N/A	N/A	N/A	MRC >3; unable to walk >100 yards	N/A	Yes, HRCT	Yes	Exhausted all medical treatment
Tutic et al,[46] 2004	>60 and lung transplant candidate or <60 and strong preference for LVRS	FEV$_1$ ≤35% of predicted	TLC >130% of predicted, RV >200% of predicted	Severe dyspnea at rest or with minimal activity	Yes	Yes	N/A	Impaired DLCO
Dauriat et al,[47] 2006	N/A	FEV$_1$ ≤40% of predicted	"TLC greater than predicted"	Yes; Fletcher dyspnea score >2	Yes	Yes, HRCT	N/A	N/A
Stoller et al,[48] 2007	N/A	FEV$_1$ <45% of predicted (≥15% of predicted if age >70 y)	TLC >100%, RV >150%	Yes; 6MWT ≥140 m after PR and able to complete 3 min of unloaded pedaling in exercise tolerance test	Yes	Yes, HRCT	N/A	BMI <31.1 kg/m^2 for males and <32.3 kg/m^2 for females; prednisone <20 mg/d, clearance from cardiology, pulmonary, thoracic surgery and anesthesiologist

(continued on next page)

150   Foray et al

Table 2
(continued)

Series	Age (y)	Severe Obstruction	Hyperinflation and Air Trapping	Severe Dyspnea	Impaired Quality of Life	Heterogeneous Emphysema on Lung Imaging	Matched V/Q Defects	Other
Tuohy et al,[49] 2011	N/A	N/A	TLC >120% of predicted, RV >180% of predicted, RV/TLC >60%	N/A	N/A	Yes, HRCT	N/A	Lobes that demonstrated marked lung destruction with an intact fissure
Hillerdal et al,[50] 2014	≤80	FEV$_1$ 15%–40% of predicted	RV >140% of predicted	Yes	Yes	Yes, CT scan	Yes	Homozygotic AATD deficiency; lack of other serious diseases
Delage et al,[51] 2019	≥40	FEV$_1$ ≤45% of predicted post-bronchodilator	TLC ≥100% of predicted, RV ≥150% of predicted	Yes; mMRC >2	N/A	Yes, HRCT	N/A	Intact fissure between target and ipsilateral lobe

Abbreviations: BMI, body mass index; CT, computed tomography; HRCT, high-resolution CT; mMRC, mMRC dyspnea scale; N/A, not applicable.

Alpha$_1$-antitrypsin Disease

Table 3
Exclusion criteria

Series	Age (y)	Active Cigarette Smoking	Pulmonary Function Test Exclusions	Paco$_2$	Bronchiectasis	Pulmonary Hypertension	Heart Disease	Cancer	Steroid Therapy	Other
Cassina et al,[44] 1998	N/A	Yes	N/A	>46 mm Hg	Yes	N/A	N/A	N/A	N/A	BMI <18 kg/m^2; ventilator-dependent; severe pleural adhesions; restrictive lung disease
Gelb et al,[45] 1999	N/A	N/A	N/A	N/A	N/A	N/A	N/A	N/A	N/A	N/A
Tutic et al,[46] 2004	>75	Yes	DLCO <20% of predicted	>55 mm Hg	Yes, or acute bronchopulmonary infection	Yes, mean PAP >35 mm Hg	CAD, HFrEF	Yes; life expectancy <2 y	>15 mg prednisolone	Vanishing lung; BMI <18 kg/m^2; addiction or psychiatric illness; relevant renal, gastrointestinal or neurologic disease
Dauriat et al,[47] 2006	>75	N/A	N/A	N/A	N/A	N/A	Yes; severe HFrEF	N/A	N/A	Giant bulla (>1/3 volume of hemithorax), BMI <18 kg/m^2

(continued on next page)

Table 3
(continued)

Series	Age (y)	Active Cigarette Smoking	Pulmonary Function Test Exclusions	Paco$_2$	Bronchiectasis	Pulmonary Hypertension	Heart Disease	Cancer	Steroid Therapy	Other
Stoller et al,[48] 2007	N/A	N/A	N/A	N/A	Yes	Yes, systolic PAP >45 mm Hg or mean PAP >35 mm Hg	Yes	N/A	N/A	Prior lung transplant, LVRS, median sternotomy or lobectomy; diffuse emphysema; weight loss >10% in 90 d; lung nodules requiring surgery; giant bulla (>1/3 volume of lung)
Tuohy et al,[49] 2011	N/A	N/A	N/A	N/A	Yes, or frequent infective exacerbations of COPD	Yes	N/A	N/A	N/A	N/A
Hillerdal et al,[50] 2014	N/A	N/A	N/A	N/A	N/A	N/A	N/A	N/A	N/A	N/A
Delage et al,[51] 2019	N/A	N/A	N/A	N/A	N/A	N/A	N/A	N/A	N/A	N/A

Abbreviations: BMI, body mass index; N/A, not applicable; PAP, pulmonary artery pressure.

Table 4
Operation characteristics

Series	Bilateral/Unilateral	Technique	Complications
Cassina et al,[44] 1998	Bilateral	Thoracotomy	1 wound hematoma requiring operative removal; pneumonia in 3 patients; delayed pneumothorax requiring repeat thoracotomy in 3 patients
Gelb et al,[45] 1999	Bilateral	VATS	ND
Tutic et al,[46] 2004	18 bilateral, 3 unilateral	VATS	Prolonged air leak >7 d in 7 patients; 5 patients underwent lung transplantation (range 3–42 mo after LVRS); 2 patients died of respiratory failure (at 24 mo and 42 mo); 1 patient committed suicide at 3 mo
Dauriat et al,[47] 2006	Unilateral	Thoracotomy	3 patients developed pneumonia/purulent bronchitis
Stoller et al,[48] 2007	Bilateral	VATS or median sternotomy	2 deaths by 24 mo
Tuohy et al,[49] 2011	Unilateral	ELVR using Zephyr valves (Pulmonx)	2 pneumothorax, 1 infective exacerbation resulting in a coughed-up valve, 1 contralateral pneumonia, 1 patient with recurrent infective exacerbations
Hillerdal et al,[50] 2014	Unilateral	ELVR using Zephyr valves (Pulmonx)	2 coughed up valves, 1 had immediate infection necessitating valve removal, 1 had repeated infection necessitating valve removal
Delage et al,[51] 2019	Unilateral	ELVR using Spiration Valve System (Olympus)	3 COPD exacerbation, 3 pneumonia, 4 pneumothorax, 1 death through 12 mo

Abbreviation: ND, no data.

improvement in FEV$_1$ at 3 months to 8 months postprocedure; 1 study did not report 3-month to 8-month data. The improvement in FEV$_1$ was on average not sustained, such that by 12 months to 24 months only 2 LRVS and 1 ELVR series reported that the FEV$_1$ remained higher than the baseline value. The results are similar for TLC and RV in that the 3-month to 8-month values for TLC and RV were meaningfully reduced in 3 of 7 series for TLC and 3 of 5 series for RV. At 12 months to 24 months, mean TLC was meaningfully reduced in none of the 4 series with data, whereas the mean RV was meaningfully decreased from baseline in 2 of 3 series. Baseline DLCO data were reported in 4 series. Follow-up DLCO data

were reported in only 3 series; 1 at 3 months to 8 months, 1 at 12 months to 24 months, and 1 at both 3 months to 8 months and 12 months to 24 months. None of the series reported a significant improvement in DLCO, although sample size is limited.

Table 6 lists the dyspnea scores at baseline, 3 months to 8 months postprocedure, and 12 months to 24 postprocedure. One series did not report dyspnea scores. In the 6 series with data at 3 months to 8 months postprocedure, 4 found a statistically significant decrease in dyspnea scores. There was a statistically significant decrease in dyspnea scores in 3 of 6 studies by 12 months to 24 months postprocedure.

Table 5
Spirometry and plethysmography values at baseline, 3 months to 8 months, and 12 months to 24 months

Series	Baseline Percent Predicted Forced Expiratory Volume in the First Second of Expiration, Mean ±SD	3-Month–8-Month Percent Predicted Forced Expiratory Volume in the First Second of Expiration, Mean ±SD	12-Month–24-Month Percent Predicted Forced Expiratory Volume in the First Second of Expiration, Mean ±SD	Baseline Percent Predicted Total Lung Capacity, Mean ±SD	3-Month–8-Month Percent Predicted Total Lung Capacity, Mean ±SD	12-Month–24-Month Percent Predicted Total Lung Capacity, Mean ± SD	Baseline Percent Predicted Residual Volume, Mean ±SD	3-Month–8-Month Percent Predicted Residual Volume, Mean ± SD	12-Month–24-Month Percent Predicted Residual Volume, Mean ±SD	Baseline Percent Predicted Diffusing Capacity for Carbon Monoxide, Mean ±SD	3-Month–8-Month Percent Predicted Diffusing Capacity for Carbon Monoxide, Mean ±SD	12-Month–24-Month Percent Predicted Diffusing Capacity for Carbon Monoxide, Mean ±SD
Cassina et al,[44] 1998	24 ± 7	38 ± 6[e]	20 ± 6	139 ± 20	114 ± 19[e]	139 ± 16	342 ± 68	254 ± 41[e]	339 ± 65	ND	ND	ND
Gelb et al,[45] 1999	30 ± 2	ND	33 ± 1	151 ± 13	ND	127 ± 10	256 ± 22	ND	181 ± 31	35 ± 9	ND	59 ± 9
Tutic et al,[46] 2004	27 ± 1.9	38 ± 3.3[e]	34 ± 3.5[e]	ND	ND	ND		ND	ND	37 ± 3	40 ± 2	43 ± 4
Dauriat et al,[47] 2006	22.2 ± 5.7	28.9 ± 11.2[e]	25.9 ± 9.1[e]	138 ± 18	132 ± 16	133 ± 20	278 ± 48	248 ± 57	259 ± 13.5	ND	ND	ND
Stoller et al,[48] 2007[a]	27.0 (26–32)	3.0 (−3–9.5)[b]	−0.5 (−3.5–5.0) [b]	129.5 (121–135)	−18.5 (−23–10.5)[c]	−15 (−21.5–6.5)[c]	216 (180–229)	−53 (−78–30)[d]	−47.5 (−64.5,-7.5)[d]	26.5 (22–38)	ND	ND
Tuohy et al,[49] 2011[a]	18.3 (14.6–21.4)	26.15 (24–30.9)[e]	ND	141.1 (131.4–152.5)	133.4 (119.3,135.2)	ND	336.3 (286–365.5)	256.8 (210–297)[e]	ND	ND	ND	ND
Hillerdal et al,[50] 2014	26 (18–34)	37 (25–64)	42 (25–80)	122 (107–141)	113 (100–130)	ND	195 (140–309)	171 (104–230)	ND	28 (25–34)	38 (35–42)	ND
Delage et al,[51] 2019	0.87 ± 0.21	0.11 ± 0.17	0.07 ± 0.18	1.83 ± 0.45	−1.16 ± 0.84	ND	ND	ND	ND	ND	ND	ND

When multiple values were reported for a given range, the highest value is listed here.
Abbreviation: ND, no data.
[a] Values reported as median (quartiles).
[b] Reported as percent change in FEV$_1$% predicted.
[c] Reported as percent change in TLC percent predicted.
[d] Reported as percent change in RV percent predicted.
[e] Statistically significant (P<.05).

Table 6
Dyspnea scores at baseline, 3 months to 8 months, and 12 months to 24 months

Series	Pre–Lung Volume Reduction Surgery Dyspnea Score, Mean ±SD (Scale Used)	3-Month–8-Month Dyspnea Score	12-Month–24-Month Maximum Improvement in Dyspnea Score
Cassina et al,[44] 1998	3.2 ± 0.6 (MRC)	1.8 ± 0.8[c]	2.2 ± 0.5[c]
Gelb et al,[45] 1999	3.2 ± 0.05 (MRC)	ND	2.2 ± 0.05
Tutic et al,[46] 2004	3.7 ± 0.1 (MRC)	1.4 ± 0.2[c]	1.7 ± 0.2[c]
Stoller et al,[48] 2007[a]	42.5 (35–54) (SGRQ)	4.6 (−11.9–6.9)[b]	10.4 (−3.7–27.3)[b]
Dauriat et al,[47] 2006	4.18 ± 0.73 (MRC)	3.1 ± 0.9[c]	3.2 ± 0.6[c]
Tuohy et al,[49] 2011[a]	4 (3,4) (MRC)	2.5 (2,3)[c]	ND
Hillerdal et al,[50] 2014	ND	ND	ND
Delage et al,[51] 2019	55.2 ± 16.0 (SGRQ)	14.3 ± 12.9	8.2 ± 12.9

When multiple values were reported for a given time range, the highest value is listed here.
   Abbreviations: MRC, MRC scale (1–5, higher scores indicate increased breathlessness); ND, no data; SGRQ, St. George's Respiratory Questionnaire (0–00, higher scores indicate more limitations).
   [a] Values reported as median (quartiles).
   [b] Reported as change in SGRQ score.
   [c] Statistically significant (*P*<.05).

Table 7 lists the 6-minute walk distance (6MWT) data at baseline, 3 months to 8 months postprocedure and 12 months to 24 months postprocedure. Five of the 7 series reported baseline and follow-up 6MWT data. The 6MWT distance was significantly improved in 3 of the 6 series at 3 months to 8 months and remained significantly improved at 12 months to 24 months in 2 of the 4 series. Patients with severe AATD showed an initial improvement following LVRS or ELVR in both PFTs and 6MWT; however, this was not sustained over 12 months to 24 months.

Table 8 lists the Pao$_2$ and Paco$_2$ data at baseline and at 3 months to 8 months and 12 months to 24 months postprocedure in the 4 series with available data. Three of the series showed statistically significant improvements in Pao$_2$ at 3 months to 8 months postprocedure; however, the absolute magnitude of the increase was not clinically important (<6 mm Hg or <0.8 kPa). Only 1 of the series reported a statistically important increase in Pao$_2$ at 12 months to 24 months, but the absolute increase likewise was clinically irrelevant (4 mm Hg or 0.53 kPa). None of the follow-up Paco$_2$ values

Table 7
Six-minute walk test at baseline, 3 months to 8 months, and 12 months to 24 months

Series	Six-Minute Walk Test, Baseline (ft), Mean ±SD	Six-Minute Walk Test, 3 Months–8 Months (ft), Mean ±SD	Six-Minute Walk Test, 12 Months–24 Months (ft), Mean ±SD
Cassina et al,[44] 1998	692 ± 338	1150[c]	985[c]
Gelb et al,[45] 1999	ND	ND	ND
Tutic et al,[46] 2004	912 ± 66	1309 ± 66[c]	1332 ± 85[c]
Dauriat et al,[47] 2006	777 ± 475	1017 ± 505[c]	885 ± 495
Stoller et al,[48] 2007[a]	1489.5 (1398–1637)	42 (−86–135)[b]	14 (−358–268.5)[b]
Tuohy et al,[49] 2011[a]	517 (344–1168)	1050 (591, 1696)	ND
Hillerdal et al,[50] 2014	ND	ND	ND
Delage et al,[51] 2019	1061	113 ± 259a	ND

When multiple values were reported for a given time range, the highest value is listed here.
   Abbreviation: ND, no data.
   [a] Values reported as median (quartiles).
   [b] Reported as change from baseline.
   [c] Statistically significant (*P*<.05).

Table 8
Arterial blood gas values at baseline, 3 months to 8 months, and 12 months to 24 months

Series	Baseline PaO$_2$, Mean ±SD (mm Hg)	PaO$_2$, 3 Months–8 Months, Mean ±SD (mm Hg)	PaO$_2$, 12 Months to 24 Months, Mean ±SD (mm Hg)	Baseline PaCO$_2$, Mean ±SD (mm Hg)	PaCO$_2$, 3 Months–8 Months, Mean ±SD (mm Hg)	PaCO$_2$, 12 Months–24 Months, Mean ±SD (mm Hg)
Cassina et al,[44] 1998	65.3 ± 7.1	69 ± 8.5[c]	67 ± 8	36.8 ± 3.3	36.5 ± 5.8	36 ± 3
Gelb et al,[45] 1999	ND	ND	ND	ND	ND	ND
Tutic et al,[46] 2004	63.6 ± 0.3	67.5 ± 0.3[c]	67.5 ± 0.2[c]	33.8 ± 0.1	36 ± 0.2	36 ± 0.1
Dauriat et al,[47] 2006	62 ± 9.7	67 ± 6.8[c]	65 ± 8.2	40 ± 6.7	38 ± 4.4	38.6 ± 4
Stoller et al,[48] 2007[a]	64.5 (58–70)	8 (–1–9.0)[b]	1 (–2–11.5)[b]	43 (42–43)	–2 (–5–3)[b]	0 (–3.5–3)[b]
Tuohy et al,[49] 2011	ND		ND	ND	ND	ND
Hillerdal et al,[50] 2014	ND	ND	ND	ND	ND	ND
Delage et al,[51] 2019	ND	ND	ND	ND	ND	ND

When multiple values were reported for a given time range, the highest value is listed here.

Abbreviation: ND, no data.

[a] Values reported as median (quartiles).
[b] Reported as change from baseline.
[c] Statistically significant ($P < .05$).

Table 9
Investigators' conclusions

Series	Conclusion
Cassina et al,[44] 1998	"In most patients with α1-protease inhibitor-deficiency emphysema, this type of surgery offers only short-term improvement in lung function, respiratory mechanics and dyspnoea, in contrast to patients with smoker's emphysema, for whom the functional improvement may be sustained for 2 yrs or longer."
Gelb et al,[45] 1999	"In summary, 2±3 yrs of follow-up of lower lobe lung volume reduction surgery in four patients with a1-antitrypsin emphysema suggests the physiological changes may be attributed to increased lung elastic recoil. Further investigative studies will be needed to define the clinical role if any of lung volume reduction surgery in a1-AT emphysema."
Tutic et al,[46] 2004	"Lung volume reduction surgery in patients with advanced emphysema from α$_1$-antitrypsin deficiency results in a significant improvement in dyspnea and lung function for as long as 3.5 years in some cases. It appears that magnitude and duration of these effects are inferior and shorter than those in patients with pure smoker's emphysema. Patients with heterogeneous disease and no or minor inflammatory airway disease may benefit most."
Dauriat et al,[47] 2006	"our experience suggests that the functional benefit is short lasting in α1-AT deficient patients who undergo unilateral LVRS for emphysema. Based on these results, we consider that LVRS remains an option but that lung transplantation, if possible, is more appropriate for most of these patients."
Stoller et al,[48] 2007	"Trends of lower magnitude and duration of FEV$_1$ rise after surgery in AATD-deficient versus AATD-replete subjects and higher mortality in deficient individuals randomized to surgery versus medical treatment suggest caution in recommending LVRS in AATD deficiency."
Tuohy et al,[49] 2011	"The data from this case series suggest that this intervention may provide bridging therapy to subsequent transplantation for younger AATD patients with end-stage emphysema."
Hillerdal et al,[50] 2014	In carefully selected AATD patients with severe emphysema, "ELVR in carefully selected AATD deficiency patients with severe emphysema can be safely performed with encouraging long-lasting results."
Delage et al,[51] 2019	"Implantation of the SVS in D patients with severe emphysema provides clinically meaningful improvements in FEV$_1$, target lobe volume reduction, quality of life parameters and exercise capacity, with an acceptable safety profile."

Abbreviation: SVS, spiration valve system.

was significantly different from baseline and all of the values were more or less in the normal range.

The authors' summary conclusions are listed in **Table 9**. The operative series acknowledged that the benefits of surgical LVRS in selected patients with severe AATD with respect to measured pulmonary function, respiratory mechanics, and exertional breathlessness were modest and short lived compared with smoker's emphysema patients with normal AATD levels. One series also reported higher mortality in the AATD group. Overall, as stated by Gelb and colleagues,[45] "the role of LVRS is uncertain" in the treatment of emphysema due to severe AATD. The 2 series that utilized unilateral endobronchial valves struck a more optimistic tone and focused on the feasibility of performing the procedure and patient safety.

SUMMARY

The improvements in measured pulmonary function, exercise capacity, and quality of life metrics for individuals with advanced emphysema due to severe AATD following LVRS are inferior, both in magnitude and duration, to the improvements seen in individuals with severe emphysema who have normal AATD levels. LVRS for patients with panacinar emphysema due to severe AATD cannot be recommended based on data from the 5 case series reviewed in this article.

CLINICS CARE POINTS

- AATD-related pulmonary emphysema largely is indistinguishable from non-AATD smoker's emphysema, making underdiagnosis and diagnostic delays common.
- All patients with COPD should be tested for AATD, regardless of smoking history.
- Treatment of AATD-related pulmonary emphysema is not significantly different than in AATD-replete patients. Smoking cessation should be emphasized, given the risk of increased rates of decline in lung function compared with AATD-replete patients.
- Intravenous augmentation therapy with purified preparations of pooled donor-derived AATD is recommended for patients with an FEV_1 in the range of 30% to 65% of predicted; augmentation therapy is debated in patients with FEV_1 less than 30% of predicted.
- Outcomes after surgical LVRS among AATD patients are inferior compared with AATD-replete patients. Surgical LVRS for AATD patients cannot be recommended based on the data from published case series.
- The role of ELVR in AATD-related pulmonary emphysema is unclear.

REFERENCES

1. Raherison C, Girodet P-O. Epidemiology of COPD. Eur Respir Rev 2009;18(114):213–21.
2. Decramer M, Janssens W, Miravitlles M. Chronic obstructive pulmonary disease. Lancet 2012; 379(9823):1341–51.
3. Rabe KF, Watz H. Chronic obstructive pulmonary disease. Lancet 2017;389(10082):1931–40.
4. Soriano JB, Polverino F, Cosio BG. What is early COPD and why is it important? Eur Respir J 2018; 52(6):1801448.
5. Wedzicha JA, Banerji D, Chapman KR, et al. Indacaterol–Glycopyrronium versus Salmeterol–Fluticasone for COPD. N Engl J Med 2016;374(23):2222–34.
6. Ferreira J, Drummond M, Pires N, et al. Optimal treatment sequence in COPD: Can a consensus be found? Rev Port Pneumol (English Ed) 2016;22(1):39–49.
7. Pavord I, Jones P, Burgel PR, et al. Exacerbations of COPD. Int J Chron Obstruct Pulmon Dis 2016;21. https://doi.org/10.2147/COPD.S85978.
8. Leuppi JD, Schuetz P, Bingisser R, et al. Short-term vs conventional glucocorticoid therapy in acute exacerbations of chronic obstructive pulmonary disease. JAMA 2013;309(21):2223.
9. Continuous or Nocturnal Oxygen Therapy in Hypoxemic Chronic Obstructive Lung Disease. Ann Intern Med 1980;93(3):391.
10. Lacasse Y, Tan A-YM, Maltais F, et al. Home Oxygen in Chronic Obstructive Pulmonary Disease. Am J Respir Crit Care Med 2018;197(10):1254–64.
11. Long term domiciliary oxygen therapy in chronic hypoxic cor pulmonale complicating chronic bronchitis and emphysema. Report of the Medical Research Council Working Party. Lancet 1981; 1(8222):681–6. Available at: http://www.ncbi.nlm.nih.gov/pubmed/6110912.
12. Sadaka A, Montgomery A, Mourad S, et al. Exercise response to oxygen supplementation is not associated with survival in hypoxemic patients with obstructive lung disease. Int J Chron Obstruct Pulmon Dis 2018;13:1607–12.
13. Lacasse Y, Sériès F, Corbeil F, et al. Randomized trial of nocturnal oxygen in chronic obstructive pulmonary disease. N Engl J Med 2020;383(12): 1129–38.
14. Rugbjerg M, Iepsen UW, Jørgensen KJ, et al. Effectiveness of pulmonary rehabilitation in COPD with mild symptoms: A systematic review with meta-analyses. Int J COPD 2015;10:791–801.
15. Rugbjerg M, Iepsen UW, Jørgensen KJ, et al. Effectiveness of pulmonary rehabilitation in COPD with mild symptoms: a systematic review with meta-analyses. Int J Chron Obstruct Pulmon Dis 2015;791. https://doi.org/10.2147/COPD.S78607.
16. Kerti M, Balogh Z, Kelemen K, et al. The relationship between exercise capacity and different functional markers in pulmonary rehabilitation for COPD. Int J Chron Obstruct Pulmon Dis 2018;13:717–24.
17. Aramburu A, Arostegui I, Moraza J, et al. COPD classification models and mortality prediction capacity. Int J Chron Obstruct Pulmon Dis 2019;14: 605–13.
18. Eriksson S. Emphysema before and after 1963 historic perspectives. COPD J Chronic Obstr Pulm Dis 2013;10(sup1):9–12.
19. Snider GL. Emphysema: the first two centuries—and beyond: a historical overview, with suggestions for future research: part 1. Am Rev Respir Dis 1992; 146(5_pt_1):1334–44.
20. Laurell CB, Eriksson S. [HYPO-ALPHA-1-ANTITRYPSINEMIA]. Verh Dtsch Ges Inn Med 1964;70:

537–9. Available at: http://www.ncbi.nlm.nih.gov/pubmed/14294270.

21. Eriksson S. Studies in alpha 1-antitrypsin deficiency. Acta Med Scand Suppl 1965;432:1–85. Available at: http://www.ncbi.nlm.nih.gov/pubmed/4160491.

22. Gross P, Babyak MA, Tolker E, et al. Enzymatically produced pulmonary emphysema; a preliminary report. J Occup Med 1964;6:481–4. Available at: http://www.ncbi.nlm.nih.gov/pubmed/14241128.

23. Strnad P, McElvaney NG, Lomas DA. Alpha1-antitrypsin deficiency. N Engl J Med 2020;382(15):1443–55.

24. de Serres F, Blanco I. Role of alpha-1 antitrypsin in human health and disease. J Intern Med 2014;276(4):311–35.

25. Janciauskiene SM, Bals R, Koczulla R, et al. The discovery of α1-antitrypsin and its role in health and disease. Respir Med 2011;105(8):1129–39.

26. Parr DG, Stoel BC, Stolk J, et al. Pattern of emphysema distribution in alpha1-antitrypsin deficiency influences lung function impairment. Am J Respir Crit Care Med 2004;170(11):1172–8.

27. Parr DG, Guest PG, Reynolds JH, et al. Prevalence and impact of bronchiectasis in alpha1-antitrypsin deficiency. Am J Respir Crit Care Med 2007;176(12):1215–21.

28. Sandhaus RA, Turino G, Brantly ML, et al. Clinical practice guidelines: The diagnosis and management of alpha-1 antitrypsin deficiency in the adult. J COPD Found 2016;3(3):668–82.

29. American Thoracic Society, European Respiratory Society. American Thoracic Society/European Respiratory Society statement: standards for the diagnosis and management of individuals with alpha-1 antitrypsin deficiency. Am J Respir Crit Care Med 2003;168(7):818–900.

30. National Emphysema Treatment Trial Research Group. A randomized trial comparing lung-volume–reduction surgery with medical therapy for severe emphysema. N Engl J Med 2003;348(21):2059–73.

31. Brantigan OC, Mueller E, Kress MB. A surgical approach to pulmonary emphysema. Am Rev Respir Dis 1959;80(1, Part 2):194–206.

32. Donahue JM, Cassivi SD. Lung volume reduction surgery for patients with alpha-1 antitrypsin deficiency emphysema. Thorac Surg Clin 2009;19(2):201–8.

33. Cooper JD, Patterson GA, Sundaresan RS, et al. Results of 150 consecutive bilateral lung volume reduction procedures in patients with severe emphysema. J Thorac Cardiovasc Surg 1996;112(5):1319–30.

34. Wood DE, DeCamp MM. The National Emphysema Treatment Trial: a paradigm for future surgical trials. Ann Thorac Surg 2001;72(2):327–9.

35. Weinmann GG, Chiang Y-P, Sheingold S. The National Emphysema Treatment Trial (NETT): a study in agency collaboration. Proc Am Thorac Soc 2008;5(4):381–4.

36. Berger RL, Wood KA, Cabral HJ, et al. Lung volume reduction surgery. Treat Respir Med 2005;4(3):201–9.

37. Banerjee S, Babidge W, Noorani H, et al. Lung volume reduction surgery for emphysema: systematic review of studies comparing different procedures [Technology report No 57]. Ottawa. 2005. Available at: https://cadth.ca/sites/default/files/pdf/176a_lvrs_tr_e.pdf.

38. Sciurba FC. Early and long-term functional outcomes following lung volume reduction surgery. Clin Chest Med 1997;18(2):259–76.

39. Martinez FJ, de Oca MM, Whyte RI, et al. Lung-volume reduction improves dyspnea, dynamic hyperinflation, and respiratory muscle function. Am J Respir Crit Care Med 1997;155(6):1984–90.

40. Ingenito EP, Loring SH, Moy ML, et al. Interpreting improvement in expiratory flows after lung volume reduction surgery in terms of flow limitation theory. Am J Respir Crit Care Med 2001;163(5):1074–80.

41. Sciurba FC, Rogers RM, Keenan RJ, et al. Improvement in pulmonary function and elastic recoil after lung-reduction surgery for diffuse emphysema. N Engl J Med 1996;334(17):1095–9.

42. LANDO Y, BOISELLE PM, SHADE D, et al. Effect of lung volume reduction surgery on diaphragm length in severe chronic obstructive pulmonary disease. Am J Respir Crit Care Med 1999;159(3):796–805.

43. BLOCH KE, LI Y, ZHANG J, et al. Effect of surgical lung volume reduction on breathing patterns in severe pulmonary emphysema. Am J Respir Crit Care Med 1997;156(2):553–60.

44. Cassina PC, Teschler H, Konietzko N, et al. Two-year results after lung volume reduction surgery in α1-antitrypsin deficiency versus smoker's emphysema. Eur Respir J 1998;12(5):1028–32.

45. Gelb AF, McKenna RJ, Brenner M, et al. Lung function after bilateral lower lobe lung volume reduction surgery for alpha1-antitrypsin emphysema. Eur Respir J 1999;14(4):928–33. Available at: http://erj.ersjournals.com/content/14/4/928.abstract.

46. Tutic M, Bloch KE, Lardinois D, et al. Long-term results after lung volume reduction surgery in patients with α1-antitrypsin deficiency. J Thorac Cardiovasc Surg 2004;128(3):408–13.

47. Dauriat G, Mal H, Jebrak G, et al. Functional results of unilateral lung volume reduction surgery in alpha1-antitrypsin deficient patients. Int J Chron Obstruct Pulmon Dis 2006;1(2):201–6.

48. Stoller JK, Gildea TR, Ries AL, et al. Lung volume reduction surgery in patients with emphysema and α-1 antitrypsin deficiency. Ann Thorac Surg 2007;83(1):241–51.

49. Tuohy MM, Remund KF, Hilfiker R, et al. Endobronchial valve deployment in severe α-1 antitrypsin

deficiency emphysema: A case series. Clin Respir J 2013;7(1):45–52.

50. Hillerdal G, Mindus S. One-to four-year follow-up of endobronchial lung volume reduction in alpha-1-antitrypsin deficiency patients: A case series. Respiration 2014;88(4):320–8.

51. Delage A, Hogarth DK, Zgoda M, et al. Endobronchial valve treatment in patients with severe emphysema due to alpha-1 antitrypsin deficiency. In: Interventional pulmonology. European Respiratory Society; 2019. p. PA4800. https://doi.org/10.1183/13993003.congress-2019.PA4800.

Postoperative Air Leaks After Lung Surgery
Predictors, Intraoperative Techniques, and Postoperative Management

Travis C. Geraci, MD*, Stephanie H. Chang, MD, Savan K. Shah, BS,
Amie Kent, MD, Robert J. Cerfolio, MD, MBA

KEYWORDS

- Lung resection • Air leak • Chest tube management • Surgical technique • Postoperative care
- Outcomes

KEY POINTS

- Air leaks after elective pulmonary resection occur in approximately 28% to 60% of patients, with most of them resolving by postoperative day four.
- Risk factors for air leak and prolonged air leak include emphysema, low forced expiratory volume in 1 second, obesity, male sex, steroid use, nutritional status, pleural adhesions, and upper lobectomy or bilobectomy.
- Intraoperative techniques such as proper tissue handling, fissure-less surgery, and select use of surgical sealants can reduce the risk of postoperative air leak.

INTRODUCTION

Postoperative air leak is one of the most common complications after pulmonary resection, occurring in 30% to 50% of patients.[1] An air leak is the egress of air from a break in the lung parenchyma or defect in a lung or bronchial staple line. Although most of the air leaks resolve spontaneously, even a minor air leak will postpone chest tube removal, contributing to prolonged postoperative pain, delayed functional status, and increased hospital length of stay. Severe or prolonged air leaks may also require intervention, including reoperation in select refractory cases.

Prevention and/or treatment of postoperative air leaks is a crucial component of perioperative care for patients undergoing pulmonary resection. This review details the management of air leaks, including predictors, intraoperative techniques, and postoperative management. Concomitant with the advancement in minimally invasive techniques for pulmonary resection, developing technologies and new enhanced recovery algorithms are challenging existing dogma regarding the management of postoperative air leak.

DEFINITIONS AND RISK FACTORS
Alveolar-Pleural Fistula

Most of the air leaks result from an alveolar-pleural fistula, which is a communication between the pulmonary parenchyma distal to a segmental bronchus and the pleural space. Alveolar-pleural fistulas are reported to occur in 28% to 60% of patients after elective, uncomplicated, pulmonary resection and are distinct from broncho-pleural fistulas.[2] Classic postoperative air leaks are described by type and size. The Robert David Cerfolio (named after RJC's father) classification system uses the traditional analog scale to codify air leaks into 4 types: forced expiratory leaks, an expiratory leak, an inspiratory leak, and a continuous

Department of Cardiothoracic Surgery, New York University Langone Health, 550 1st Avenue, 15th Floor, New York, NY 10016, USA
* Corresponding author.
E-mail address: travis.geraci@nyulangone.org

Thorac Surg Clin 31 (2021) 161–169
https://doi.org/10.1016/j.thorsurg.2021.02.005
1547-4127/21/© 2021 Elsevier Inc. All rights reserved.

air leak.[3] Forced expiratory leaks are those leaks elicited during patient coughing. Current digital systems are now able to quantify air leaks to double digit (Thopaz, Medela, Barr, Switzerland) or single digit mL/min (Thoraguard, Centese, Omaha, NE, USA) (**Fig. 1**).

Risk Factors for Air Leak

Numerous risk factors contribute to the development of air leaks. The most consistent risk factor is chronic obstructive pulmonary disease (COPD), with a strong correlation between the degree of emphysema and risk of developing an air leak.[4] Specifically, reduced preoperative forced expiratory volume in 1 second (FEV_1) and reduced FEV_1/forced vital capacity ratio are significant predictors of air leak.[5,6] The incidence of air leak is highest in patients with an FEV_1 less than 70%. Other risk factors include steroid use, smoking history, male sex, pleural adhesions, and decreased carbon monoxide lung diffusion capacity (DLCO).[7] Patients undergoing a lobectomy— compared with a wedge resection or segmentectomy—have a higher risk of air leak, specifically a right upper lobectomy or bilobectomy.[5,7] In a study by Isowa and colleagues,[8] poor nutritional status, indicated by low serum albumin and cholinesterase, was predictive of air leak.

Prolonged Air Leak

Most air leaks (26%–48%) will spontaneously resolve by the morning of postoperative day (POD) 1, with most of the air leaks resolving by POD 5.[9–11] In up to 6% to 18% of patients, the air leak may fail to resolve within 5 days, which the Society of Thoracic Surgeons (STS) defines as a prolonged air leak (PAL). At our institution, given the reduction of postoperative length of stay with minimally invasive techniques, we consider any air leak that delays hospital discharge as "prolonged," regardless of the number of PODs. PAL can be the result of a sizable

injury to the lung parenchyma/airway or delayed adherence of the visceral pleura to the parietal pleura due to lower postresection lung volume that is unable to fill the hemithorax. PAL is associated with increased length of stay, increased cost, increased incidence of empyema, readmission, and other postoperative complications.[12] Following lung volume reduction surgery (LVRS), the incidence of PAL is significantly higher and often prolonged for a much longer duration.[13]

Risk Factors for Prolonged Air Leak

Air leaks on POD 1 with a higher likelihood of becoming PALs are those with higher volumes of air loss (grade 4 or greater), expiratory in nature, and leaks associated with pneumothorax.[9] Using a cohort of patients with a PAL rate of 8.6%, Attaar and colleagues[14] formulated a prediction model for PAL with 76% accuracy. The model also stratifies patients into low-, intermediate-, and high-risk categories, with a PAL rate of 2%, 8.8%, and 19%, respectively. The prediction nomogram scored risk factors, including FEV_1, procedure type, smoking status, Zubrod score, preoperative hospitalization, reoperation, and procedures via thoracotomy. In an STS General Thoracic Database cohort of 50,000 patients after lung resection for lung cancer, the rate of PAL was 10.4%. On multivariate analysis, Seder and colleagues[15] determined that increased body mass index, lobectomy or bilobectomy, FEV_1 less than or equal to 70%, male sex, and right upper lobe procedures are risk factors, with their risk model correctly classifying 79% of patients at high- or low-risk of PAL.

INTRAOPERATIVE MANAGEMENT
Assessment of Air Leak

The most common method for the intraoperative evaluation of air leak is the submersion test. The chest is filled with saline and the operative lung is ventilated, with air bubbles identifying sources

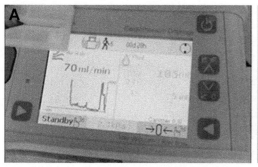
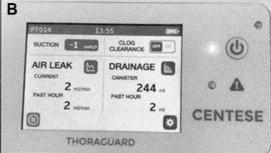

Fig. 1. Interface display of digital drainage systems. (*A*) Thopaz system demonstrating a 70 mL/min air leak. (*B*) Thoraguard system, demonstrating a 2 mL/min air leak.

of air leak. Air leaks can also be quantified by assessment of tidal volume loss on the ventilator. Tidal volume loss can be separated into mild (<100 mL/min), moderate (100–400 mL/min), or severe (>400 mL/min). Mild leaks are often self-limited and not treated, whereas severe air leaks should be reexplored. After lung resection, if a patient is difficult to ventilate at closure and there is a large air leak, the chest tube should be taken off suction while on positive ventilation. Once extubated, the tube can be returned to suction as clinically indicated.

Prevention of Air Leak

Several surgical strategies help prevent air leaks. The most important approach is appropriate tissue handling to avoid parenchymal tearing during tissue manipulation and retraction. Not enough can be said about this if fissure diving is used. The robotic platform allows a magnified view of the fissure, which can help identify where one lobe starts and another lobe ends. If early chest tube removal is planned, meticulous technique in the fissure is required. In addition, the use of fissure-less dissection has been reported to result in decreased incidence and severity of air leaks in patients with fused or incomplete fissures.[16] Traditionally, exposure of the pulmonary artery occurs with dissection at the fissure. However, in the fissure-less technique, the lung parenchyma is divided using surgical staplers after the separation of the lobar bronchus, in order to reduce the potential air leak,[17] which often entails dissection posteriorly to identify the bronchus and/or artery from the back.

During a minimally invasive pulmonary resection, it is imperative to avoid puncturing the lung during initial port placement. Despite single lung ventilation, the lung may remain adherent to the chest wall by physiologic pleural apposition or from pleural adhesions secondary to prior surgery, tube thoracostomy, neoadjuvant therapy, or an inflammatory pleural process. If a puncture occurs, the defect should be repaired with an interrupted suture (**Fig. 2**). After the initial trocar is placed, the remaining ports or incisions should be placed under direct visualization.

Treatment of Air Leak

When air leaks are identified during pulmonary resection, several operative techniques may help decrease air leak severity and duration.

Increased pleural-pleural apposition
Obliteration of the pleural space reduces the potential of air leak, by increasing pleural-pleural

apposition. Pulmonary mobilization by lysis of intrapleural adhesions, division of the inferior pulmonary ligament, and/or incising the mediastinal pleura may help the lung achieve pleural apposition. An apical pleural tent, which is performed by releasing the apical parietal pleura from the endothoracic fascia circumferentially, allows the parietal pleural to drape over and adhere to the remaining lung. This technique creates a small cavity with a fully drained space.[18] In a prospective randomized study of 48 patients with COPD undergoing right upper lobectomy, a pleural tent was performed in 23 patients with reduced incidence, severity, and duration of air leak, albeit with a significantly higher volume of pleural drainage in the pleural tent cohort.[19] However, in this trial, there was no difference in overall chest tube duration or hospital length of stay.

For patients undergoing a right middle lobe and lower lobe bilobectomy, creation of pneumoperitoneum at the time of surgery has been reported as a strategy to reduce the residual pleural space. At the time of operation, 1200 mL of air is injected under the right hemidiaphragm through a small diaphragmatic opening. Cerfolio and colleagues[20] demonstrated this method to be safe, reporting decreased incidence of air leaks and pneumothoraces, thereby shortening hospital length of stay. This method is not routinely used but can be considered with patients with minimal residual lung. Our current practice is to treat the bilobectomy space similar to a lobectomy: placement of a chest tube, with or without the application of a surgical sealant.

Surgical sealants
Surgical sealants, such as glues or patches, can be applied along the visceral pleural surface and

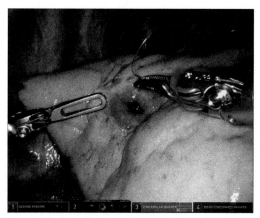

Fig. 2. Suture repair (3-0 nonabsorbable suture) of a lung laceration of the left lower lobe sustained during insertion of the initial robotic trocar.

parenchymal staple lines to prevent or reduce air leak. However, the efficacy of surgical sealants is mixed. In a 2010 Cochrane Database Review assessing 16 randomized trials, most of the studies demonstrated significant prevention or reduction of postoperative air leak, but only 3 trials reported a significant reduction in time to chest tube removal.[21] Similarly, a clear association between the use of sealants and hospital length of stay was not established, with only 3 trials demonstrating decreased hospital length of stay by a median of 1.5 days with the use of surgical sealants. In a meta-analysis of 13 trials, the use of surgical sealants had a statistically significant pooled effect size of 0.55 for reducing PAL (defined in the trials as greater than 7 days).[22] Despite these positive findings, the investigators warn that the results "should be interpreted with caution," given the heterogeneity of the studies and publication bias of those selected for analysis.

At our institution, we do not routinely use sealants. However, in select high-risk patients with wide patches of denuded or injured visceral pleura or if a minor leak is visualized from the parenchymal staple line, we use Progel (Neomend, Irvine CA). Progel is unique among sealants, as it conforms to the lung tissue, allowing expansion and relaxation without dislodging the sealant. For patients with an identified intraoperative air leak, Progel has been shown to reduce the number of patients with air leak and decrease hospital length stay.[23] The ability of Progel to seal an air leak correlated to the severity of the leak.

CHEST TUBES AND MANAGEMENT OF AIR LEAKS

Chest tubes are placed after pulmonary resection to drain fluid and/or air from the pleural space. Chest tube drainage helps maintain visceral-to-parietal pleural apposition while decreasing postoperative effusion and pneumothoraces. Our current practice is placement of a single straight 24 or 28 Fr chest tube posteriorly to the apex of the chest, with routine use of a digital drainage system. If no leak is present and the postoperative radiograph reveals a fully expanded lung, the chest tube is removed on the day of surgery, regardless of fluid output. Patients routinely have a high fat meal (usually ice cream) before removal as a provocative test for chylothorax. Chest tube removal is performed at end of expiration, which has a lower incidence of nonclinically significant pneumothorax than at end of inspiration.[24]

It is important to distinguish true air leaks from false air leaks. In patients with large or continuous air leaks, the chest tube, tubing, and drainage system should be evaluated for loose connections or breaks, which may result in the "air leak." To test for a system leak, the chest tube should be clamped at the chest wall. If air continues to leak and there is no hole in the chest tube, the drainage system should be replaced. In addition, in patients with a fixed pleural space deficit due to low-volume residual lung parenchyma, a small volume of air may be expressed through the chest tube with forced expiration, mimicking an air leak.[10] A clamp trial—where the chest tube is clamped for 2 to 4 hours with assessment for dyspnea and obtaining a chest radiograph to determine the stability or progression of pneumothorax—helps differentiate a fixed space versus a true air leak.

Reviewing 153 robotic anatomic pulmonary resections, we have discharged 12% of patients home with a chest tube and digital drainage device on POD 1 with a median duration of 4 days until the chest tube is removed in clinic.[25] In patients with a leak that does not resolve after 2 weeks, the chest tube may still be removed, even with a concomitant pneumothorax. In a retrospective study by Cerfolio and colleagues,[26] 199 patients (3.8%) were discharged home with a chest tube after pulmonary resection. After a median of 16 days, 57 patients had their chest tube removed while still having an air leak, including 26 with a nonexpanding pneumothorax. We believe chest tube removal in patients with an air leak is safe, provided they are asymptomatic, have no subcutaneous emphysema, and there is no increase in the pleural space deficit. Prophylactic antibiotics are recommended in order to avoid empyema.

Avoiding Chest Tubes

With a focus on enhanced recovery, select surgeons have questioned the necessity of postoperative chest tubes after elective pulmonary resection. Chest tubes after pulmonary resection increase pain, reduce pulmonary and functional capacity, and increase hospital length of stay. Several studies have revealed that omitting chest tubes after minimally invasive pulmonary wedge resection is feasible and safe.[27,28] In these trials, the rate of postoperative pneumothorax was 10% to 13.3%, but no patients required chest tube placement. In 162 patients who underwent thoracoscopic anatomic lung resection, Murakami and colleagues[29] identified intraoperative air leaks with a water submersion test in 112 (69%) patients and sealed them with a combination of bioabsorbable mesh and fibrin glue. After confirming no air leak after extubation, the chest tube was removed in the operating room in 102 patients (91%). No patients required placement of a chest tube for subsequent air leak or pleural effusion. In another study by Ueda and colleagues,[30] a postoperative chest tube was omitted in 53 patients (46%) after minimally invasive anatomic lung resection, with associated reduction in pain and analgesic use and improvement in pulmonary and functional capacity. Of note, these trials did not include patients undergoing LVRS, and the practice of omitting a postoperative chest tube in these patients is not recommended due to the high incidence of air leak.

Digital Drainage Systems

The use of digital chest tube drainage systems has advanced the management of air leak by introducing the advantages of objective assessment, continuous data gathering, and portability. Digital systems record air leak and pleural fluid volumes accurately and are able to adjust levels of suction with precision. Most notably, the objective nature of these systems reduces interobserver variability, allowing all members of the team to accurately assess an air leak. Digital systems also collect data continuously, allowing interpretation of data trends over time and can capture of intermittent leaks.

In prospective trials, the use of digital drainage systems has reduced the duration of chest tubes and decreased hospital length of stay when compared with traditional analog systems.[31–33] Earlier removal of chest tubes is associated with improved pulmonary function, reduced postoperative pain, and fewer overall complications.[32–34] The use of digital drainage systems are also associated with superior patient satisfaction, including the ability to ambulate and convenience of use in the outpatient setting.

The threshold volume of air leak for chest tube removal differs across trials from 0 mL/min to 50 mL/min, over a period of 6 to 12 hours. In our practice, we use 20 mL/min as signifying resolution of air leak and routinely remove chest tubes at this level. In patients with a low-grade volume loss of 10 to 20 mL/min, before removal, we perform a provocative test, which can determine the presence or absence of air leak: the system suction is increased to 40 to 60 mm Hg, with the volume increasing to approximately 50 to 100 mL/min while evacuating the pleural space. After 20 to 30 seconds, the volume of air leak will then reduce to 0 mL/min, indicating no air leak, or will stay greater than zero (10–30 mL/min), indicating the presence of an air leak.

Data trends on digital systems can also guide chest tube management. In a cohort of patients undergoing pulmonary resection with a 5.8% rate

of PAL, Takamochi and colleagues[35] reported that the incidence of PAL was significantly higher in patients with a peak air leak greater than or equal to 100 mL/min compared with less than 100 mL/min. Furthermore, they described 2 patterns of air leak over the initial 72 hours after surgery that are associated with PAL: repeated exacerbation and remission of air leak and an air leak without a progressive trend toward improvement.

POSTOPERATIVE INTERVENTIONS FOR AIR LEAK

There are several interventional treatment options to address a prolonged air leak.[4] Although our preference is to manage the pleural space using outpatient chest tubes, other options include chemical pleurodesis, autologous blood patch, placement of endobronchial valves, or reoperative strategies including topical sealants or focal wedge resection, which can be combined with chemical or mechanical pleurodesis (**Fig. 3**). More aggressive surgical strategies, such as muscle-flap obliteration of the pleural space or omentopexy, are often unnecessary for standard PAL and more frequently used for management of bronchopleural fistulas.

Pleurodesis

Instillation of a sclerosing agent into the pleural space promotes pleural apposition by forming inflammatory adhesions, leading to air leak closure. Chemical pleurodesis is used selectively in patients with a significantly prolonged air leak (greater than 20 days) in the context of a well-positioned chest tube and/or when the lung drops significantly when placed to water seal. Several agents have shown to be effective, including tetracycline, doxycycline, and talc, with success rates between 60% and 90%.[5] Successful pleurodesis via a chest tube requires pleural symphysis; therefore, chemical pleurodesis may not be effective in patients with a large pleural deficit or pneumothorax.

Blood Patch

Although at our institution, we do not perform an autologous blood patch for air leak, this method has shown success in resolving PAL in several small prospective studies. In a randomized trial, 10 patients with PAL after lobectomy were randomized to treatment with a blood patch: instillation of 120 mL of autologous blood via an apical chest drain and repeated if necessary.[36] Air leaks were sealed within 24 hours of blood patch instillation in 60% of patients, with significant reductions

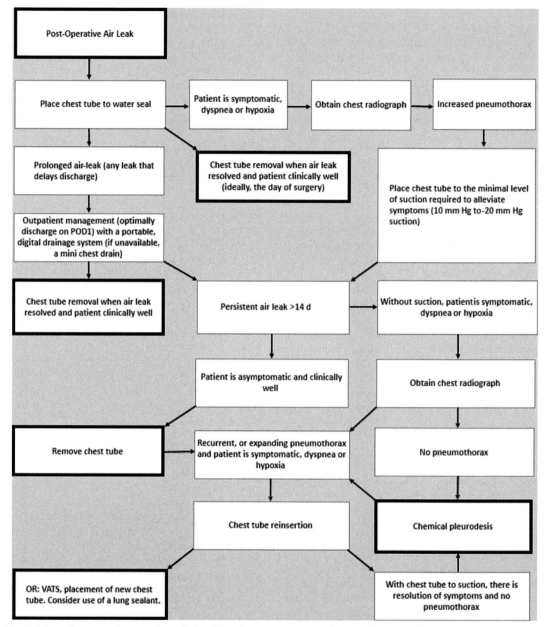

Fig. 3. Flow diagram of our preferred algorithm for management of a postoperative air leak from an aleveolar-pleural fistula. Of note, this management plan is not applicable for a segmental or bronchopleural fistula.

in chest tube dwell time and hospital length of stay. Periprocedural antibiotics have been suggested to decrease pleural contamination and reduce the incidence of empyema, which occurred in one patient (10%). A larger volume of blood seems to be more effective than smaller dose, as shown by Andretti and colleagues[37] in a randomized trial. Twenty-five patients were assigned to a 50 mL or 100 mL blood patch, with resolved air leak in 2.3 days versus 1.5 days postprocedure, respectively.

Endobronchial Valves

Patients with severe PAL or leaks refractory to other methods of control may benefit from bronchoscopic placement of a unidirectional endobronchial valve (EBV) in the segmental bronchi, occluding distal airflow while allowing drainage of secretions and trapped air. Distal parenchymal atelectasis induces tissue apposition and subsequent healing of parenchymal defects. In a series of 7 patients, Gillespie and colleagues[38] demonstrated the safety and feasibility of EBV placement in patients with a median duration of air leak of 4 weeks. All patients had a reduction in air leak, with a mean duration of 4.5 days until resolution. Discharge within 2 to 3 days was achieved in 57% of patients, and all valves were eventually removed without procedural or valve-related complications. In a series of 21 patients, Reed and colleagues[39] reported that EBV placement resulted in a median duration of chest tube removal of 15 days and a median length of stay of 5 days. For the postoperative air leak cohort (8 patients), the median length of stay was 3 days after EBV, with a mean valve dwell time of 47 days until removal.

AIR LEAK AFTER LUNG VOLUME REDUCTION SURGERY

LVRS is a palliative procedure for select patients with severe emphysema and can lead to significant functional improvement.[40,41] Emphysematous lung parenchyma is associated with increased postoperative air leaks, with up to 90% of LVRS patients in the National Emphysema Treatment Trial (NETT) experiencing an air leak within 30 days of surgery.[40] Ciccone and colleagues[41] noted that among 250 patients, PAL (>7 days) occurred in 45% (n = 113) patients, with 3.2% (n = 8) requiring reexploration for air leaks. A study evaluating postoperative air leaks in NETT showed a median air leak duration of 7 days, with increased air leak duration associated with lower DLCO, pleural adhesions, predominantly upper lobe disease, inhaled steroid usage, and Caucasians.[13] Although there was no difference in mortality for patients who experienced air leak after LVRS versus those who did not, patients with air leaks were more likely to have postoperative pneumonia and admission to the intensive care unit.

Given the high rate of postoperative air leaks following LVRS, many methods have been used in an attempt to prevent this complication. Analysis of NETT demonstrated that development of postoperative air leak was not affected by use of pleural tents, fibrin glue, or concurrent chemical pleurodesis.[13] In a randomized prospective study, Moser and colleagues[42] evaluated 25 patients who underwent bilateral LVRS, with fibrin sealant placed on the staple lines on one side and no intervention on the other side. PAL was decreased in the treatment group (4.5% treated vs 31.8% untreated), as was mean chest tube duration (2.8 days treated vs 5.9 days untreated). Reported by Tacconi and colleagues,[43] unilateral plication of the most emphysematous lung parenchyma under epidural anesthesia is another proposed technique to reduce air leak during LVRS. In this study, the plication group had

a lower incidence of PAL (18% vs 40%), shorter air leak duration (5.2 days vs 7.9 days), and shorter hospital stay (6.3 days vs 9.2 days) when compared with the traditional resection group.

SUMMARY

Alveolar air leaks after pulmonary resection remain a common complication, increasing postoperative complications and length of hospital stay. Developing technologies such as digital drainage systems combined with enhanced recovery pathways of care, however, are moving the management of air leak to the outpatient setting. Further study is warranted to define the role of avoiding chest tubes for patients after pulmonary resection.

CLINICS CARE POINTS

- Air leak after elective pulmonary resection occurs in 28% to 60% of patients and are more likely to develop in patients with limited pulmonary function (low FEV1), obesity, steroid use or immunosuppression, malnutrition, and in those undergoing an upper lobe lobectomy.

- Intraoperative techniques such as proper tissue handling, fissureless surgery, and the select use of surgical sealants can reduce the risk of postoperative air leak.

- Most of the postoperative air leaks will resolve with chest tube drainage alone by POD 4. There are several methods to address an air leak that persists beyond 5 days, including outpatient chest tube management and chemical pleurodesis.

- Digital drainage systems offer several advantages over analog systems such as an accurate digital interface, portability with suction, and precision adjustment of settings. Digital drainage systems have shown to limit interobserver variability regarding decision-making for chest tube management and had equally shown to reduce length of stay after pulmonary resection.

- LVRS for select patients with severe emphysema has a high rate of postoperative air leak (up to 90%). Using a buttressed technique and/or surgical fibrin sealants have both shown to reduce the rate of postoperative air leak in this population.

DISCLOSURE

Dr T.C. Geraci, Mr S.K. Shah, Dr S.H. Chang, and Dr A. Kent have no disclosures. Dr R.J. Cerfolio discloses past relationships with AstraZeneca, Bard Davol, Bovie Medical Corporation, C-SATS, ConMed, Covidien/Medtronic, Ethicon, Fruit Street Health, Google/Verb Surgical, Intuitive Surgical, KCI/Acelity, Myriad Genetics, Neomend, Pinnacle Biologics, ROLO-7, Tego, and TransEnterix.

REFERENCES

1. Okereke I, Murthy SC, Alster JM, et al. Characterization and Importance of Air Leak After Lobectomy. Ann Thorac Surg 2005;79(4):1167–73.
2. Alphonso N, Tan C, Utley M, et al. A prospective randomized controlled trial of suction versus non-suction to the under-water seal drains following lung resection. Eur J Cardiothorac Surg 2005;27(3):391–4.
3. Cerfolio RJ. Advances in thoracostomy tube management. Surg Clin North Am 2002;121:831–5.
4. Singhal S, Ferraris VA, Bridges CR, et al. Management of alveolar air leaks after pulmonary resection. Ann Thorac Surg 2010;89(4):1327–35.
5. Liberman M, Muzikansky A, Wright CD, et al. Incidence and risk factors of persistent air leak after major pulmonary resection and use of chemical pleurodesis. Ann Thorac Surg 2010;89(3):891–8.
6. Rivera C, Bernard A, Falcoz PE, et al. Characterization and prediction of prolonged air leak after pulmonary resection: a nationwide study setting up the index of prolonged air leak. Ann Thorac Surg 2011;92(3):1062–8.
7. Brunelli A, Cassivi SD, Halgren L. Risk factors for prolonged air leak after pulmonary resection. Thorac Surg Clin 2010;20(3):359–64.
8. Isowa N, Hasegawa S, Bando T, et al. Preoperative risk factors for prolonged air leak following lobectomy or segmentectomy for primary lung cancer. Eur J Cardiothorac Surg 2002;21(5):951.
9. Brunelli A, Monteverde M, Borri A, et al. Predictors of prolonged air leak after pulmonary lobectomy. Ann Thorac Surg 2004;77(4):1205–10.
10. Cerfolio RJ, Tummala RP, Holman WL, et al. A prospective algorithm for the management of air leaks after pulmonary resection. Ann Thorac Surg 1998;66(5):1726–30.
11. Cerfolio RJ, Bass C, Katholi CR. Prospective randomized trial compares suction versus water seal for air leaks. Ann Thorac Surg 2001;71(5):1613–7.
12. Liang S, Ivanovic J, Gilbert S, et al. Quantifying the incidence and impact of postoperative prolonged alveolar air leak after pulmonary resection. J Thorac Cardiovasc Surg 2013;145(4):948–54.
13. DeCamp MM, Blackstone EH, Naunheim KS, et al. Patient and surgical factors influencing air leak after lung volume reduction surgery: lessons learned from the national emphysema treatment trial. Ann Thorac Surg 2006;82(1):197–207.
14. Attaar A, Winger DG, Luketich JD, et al. A clinical prediction model for prolonged air leak after pulmonary resection. J Thorac Cardiovasc Surg 2017;153(3):690–9.e2.
15. Seder CW, Basu S, Ramsay T, et al. A prolonged air leak score for lung cancer resection: an analysis of the Society of Thoracic Surgeons General Thoracic Surgery Database. Ann Thorac Surg 2019;108(5):1478–83.
16. Gómez-Caro A, Calvo MJ, Lanzas JT, et al. The approach of fused fissures with fissureless technique decreases the incidence of persistent air leak after lobectomy. Eur J Cardiothorac Surg 2007;31(2):203–8.
17. Temes RT, Willms CD, Endara SA, et al. Fissureless lobectomy. Ann Thorac Surg 1998;65(1):282–4.
18. Burt BM, Shrager JB. The prevention and management of air leaks following pulmonary resection. Thorac Surg Clin 2015;25(4):411–9.
19. Allama AM. Pleural tent for decreasing air leak following upper lobectomy: a prospective randomized trial. Eur J Cardiothorac Surg 2010;38(6):674–8.
20. Cerfolio RJ, Holman WL, Katholi CR. Pneumoperitoneum after concomitant resection of the right middle and lower lobes (bilobectomy). Ann Thorac Surg 2000;70(3):942–7.
21. Belda-Sanchís J, Serra-Mitjans M, Iglesias Sentis M, et al. Surgical sealant for preventing air leaks after pulmonary resections in patients with lung cancer. Cochrane Database Syst Rev 2010;2010(1):CD003051.
22. Malapert G, Hanna HA, Pages PB, et al. Surgical sealant for the prevention of prolonged air leak after lung resection: meta-analysis. Ann Thorac Surg 2010;90(6):1779–85.
23. Allen MS, Wood DE, Hawkinson RW, et al. Prospective randomized study evaluating a biodegradable polymeric sealant for sealing intraoperative air leaks that occur during pulmonary resection. Ann Thorac Surg 2004;77(5):1792–801.
24. Cerfolio RJ, Bryant AS, Skylizard L, et al. Optimal technique for the removal of chest tubes after pulmonary resection. J Thorac Cardiovasc Surg 2013;145(6):1535–9.
25. Geraci TC, Chang SH, Ferrari-Light D, et al. Discharging Patients on Postoperative Day One after Robotic Anatomic Pulmonary Resection. Accepted abstract to the WTSA, 2020.
26. Cerfolio RJ, Minnich DJ, Bryant AS. The removal of chest tubes despite an air leak or a pneumothorax. Ann Thorac Surg 2009;87(6):1690–6.
27. Zhang JT, Dong S, Chu XP, et al. Randomized trial of an improved drainage strategy versus routine chest tube after lung wedge resection. Ann Thorac Surg 2020;109(4):1040–6.
28. Yang SM, Wang ML, Hung MH, et al. Tubeless uniportal thoracoscopic wedge resection for

peripheral lung nodules. Ann Thorac Surg 2017;
103(2):462–8.

29. Murakami J, Ueda K, Tanaka T, et al. The validation of a no-drain policy after thoracoscopic major
lung resection. Ann Thorac Surg 2017;104(3):
1005–11.

30. Ueda K, Haruki T, Murakami J, et al. No drain after
thoracoscopic major lung resection for cancer helps
preserve the physical function. Ann Thorac Surg
2019;108(2):399–404.

31. Bertolaccini L, Rizzardi G, Filice MJ, et al. 'Six sigma
approach' - an objective strategy in digital assessment of postoperative air leaks: a prospective randomised study. Eur J Cardiothorac Surg 2011;39(5):
e128–32.

32. Cerfolio RJ, Bryant AS. The benefits of continuous
and digital air leak assessment after elective pulmonary resection: a prospective study. Ann Thorac
Surg 2008;86(2):396–401.

33. Pompili C, Detterbeck F, Papagiannopoulos K, et al.
Multicenter international randomized comparison of
objective and subjective outcomes between elec-
tronic and traditional chest drainage systems. Ann
Thorac Surg 2014;98(2):490–7.

34. Miller DL, Helms GA, Mayfield WR. Digital drainage
system reduces hospitalization after video-assisted
thoracoscopic surgery lung resection. Ann Thorac
Surg 2016;102(3):955–61.

35. Takamochi K, Imashimizu K, Fukui M, et al. Utility of
objective chest tube management after pulmonary
resection using a digital drainage system. Ann
Thorac Surg 2017;104(1):275–83.

36. Shackcloth MJ, Poullis M, Jackson M, et al. Intrapleural instillation of autologous blood in the treatment of prolonged air leak after lobectomy: a
prospective randomized controlled trial. Ann Thorac
Surg 2006;82(3):1052–6.

37. Andreetti C, Venuta F, Anile M, et al. Pleurodesis with
an autologous blood patch to prevent persistent air
leaks after lobectomy. J Thorac Cardiovasc Surg
2007;133(3):759–62.

38. Gillespie CT, Sterman DH, Cerfolio RJ, et al. Endobronchial valve treatment for prolonged air leaks of the lung:
a case series. Ann Thorac Surg 2011;91(1):270–3.

39. Reed MF, Gilbert CR, Taylor MD, et al. Endobronchial Valves for Challenging Air Leaks. Ann Thorac
Surg 2015;100(4):1181–6.

40. Fishman A, Martinez F, Naunheim K, et al.
A randomized trial comparing lung-volume-reduction
surgery with medical therapy for severe emphysema.
N Engl J Med 2003;348:2059–73.

41. Ciccone AM, Meyers BF, Guthrie TG, et al. Long-
term outcome of bilateral lung volume reduction in
250 consecutive patients. J Thorac Cardiovasc
Surg 2003;125:513–25.

42. Moser C, Opitz I, Zhai W, et al. Autologous fibrin
sealant reduces the incidence of prolonged air
leak and duration of chest tube drainage after lung
volume reduction surgery: a prospective randomized blinded study. J Thorac Cardiovasc Surg
2008;136:843–9.

43. Tacconi F, Pompeo E, Mineo TC. Duration of air leak is
reduced after awake nonresectional lung volume reduction surgery. Eur J Cardiothorac Surg 2009;35:822–8.

Value of a Multidisciplinary Team Approach to Treatment of Emphysema

Sean C. Wightman, MD[a], Robert J. McKenna Jr, MD[b,c],*

KEYWORDS

- LVRS • Lung volume reduction surgery • National emphysema treatment trial (NETT)

KEY POINTS

- Successful lung volume reduction surgery (LVRS) requires a well-organized multidisciplinary team effort.
- The multidiscipline team should include the lung transplant team to help decide if the best treatment for the patient would be LVRS or lung transplant.
- LVRS is potentially indicated for patients who are symptomatic despite maximal medical management for bullous emphysema.
- Patients for LVRS have severe obstructive disease (forced expiratory volume in 1 second 20%–40% predicted, total lung volume >120%, and residual volume >120%) and a heterogeneous pattern of emphysema.

INTRODUCTION

Lung volume reduction surgery (LVRS) can greatly improve the quality of life for patients with failed medical management for severe emphysema. Chronic obstructive pulmonary disease is a leading cause of death in the western world with at least 2 million patients with emphysema.[1] Very intensive work is required for the evaluation and treatment of these patients. These patients have extremely poor pulmonary function and conditioning so their treatment carries substantial risk.

The pathophysiology behind emphysema is the loss of elastic recoil of the lungs leading to frequent air trapping in increase in the nonfunctional portions of the lung.[1] The elastic recoil of the lungs is poor,[2] such that they do not decompress well with expiration. The lung remains hyperexpanded and the diaphragm is flattened and very low in the chest; it cannot move. LVRS was developed to remove the nonfunctioning portions of the lung, those simply occupying space, making more physical space within the chest for the portions of the lung with continued function.[1] The basic physiology behind LVRS is to improve the elastic recoil of the emphysematous lung. Patients with severe emphysema have high TLC (total lung capacity) and the RV (residual volume) is high so the diaphragm is low in the chest. The total elastic recoil is the average of the recoil if all areas of the lung. If the lung is uniformly bad (homogeneous), resection of some of that bad tissue does not generally improve the recoil because the average elastic recoil does not improve. The optimal scenario is a heterogeneous pattern of

Conflict of Interest: The authors report no potential conflicts of interest.

Funding: This article had no outside funding sources.

a Division of Thoracic Surgery, Keck School of Medicine, The University of Southern California, Los Angeles, CA, USA; b Department of Surgery, John Wayne Cancer Institute, Los Angeles, CA, USA; c Thoracic Surgery, Stanford University

* Corresponding author. 400 South Windsor, Los Angeles, CA 90020.

E-mail address: Robert.mckenna@providence.org

Thorac Surg Clin 31 (2021) 171–175

https://doi.org/10.1016/j.thorsurg.2021.02.004

emphysema, where the lungs have bad, nonfunctional areas of lung tissue and some better areas. By removing the bad areas, the better areas can expand and function more effectively. Removing bad areas of lung with poor elastic recoil increases the overall average of recoil for the whole lung so breathing improves. The RV is better. The diaphragm is higher in the chest and can function much better because it can move caudally with inspiration. LVRS is performed in patients with a heterogeneous pattern of emphysema.[3,4]

Although initially reported by Brantigan and Mueller,[5] this was popularized by Cooper and colleagues[6] when they reported on a series of 20 patients using a linear stapler to cut out the bad tissue. The National Emphysema Treatment Trial (NETT) validated this technique, especially for patients with upper lobe emphysema predominance[3] and demonstrated its durability.[7] Importantly, the NETT also highlighted patient risk factors where LVRS should be avoided.[3,7] To avoid mortality due to poor patient selection and postoperative complications, multidisciplinary teams for LVRS are a key to success and the foundation of any LVRS program.[8]

Here, we have been tasked to discuss the importance of the LVRS multidisciplinary team approach to treatment of emphysema.

INTRODUCTION TO THE TEAM

The pulmonary medicine and thoracic surgery divisions are the core of the LVRS multidisciplinary team. At some institutions, a combination multidisciplinary clinic, consolidating patient visits, is offered to provide consults and testing (eg, plethysmography, computerized tomography [CT] scan, as well as a radionuclide perfusion scan).[1] Team meetings discuss patients and appropriate plans for each. The core composition includes pulmonologists, thoracic surgeons, radiologists, physical therapists, and an LVRS coordinator. Other important team members include the immediate postoperative care team composed of anesthesiologists, nurses, and respiratory therapists.

LUNG VOLUME REDUCTION SURGERY COORDINATOR

The quality of an LVRS program is greatly enhanced by a high-functioning coordinator. In the middle of the 1990s, our LVRS program was very busy with approximately 8 operations per week. The coordinator streamlines screening and evaluation processes.[8] In our program, we required, at a minimum, a medical history, pulmonary function test, and CT scan to identify potential candidates for the procedures. Documentation of

consensus recommendations by the multidisciplinary team is also a fundamental role of the LVRS coordinator.[8] Oey and Waller[8] described a documentation form used to standardize information and keep it readily accessible with completion being the role of the coordinator. If they appeared to be good candidates, they then came to our clinic for an in-person evaluation. Our coordinator was extremely busy in the process of organizing these extensive evaluations, coordinating the evaluations of the information mailed to us, organizing clinic visits, and during their subsequent operation if they were deemed appropriate candidates.

PULMONOLOGIST

A pulmonologist is important for helping to screen potential patients and perioperative care. The pulmonologist needs to make sure that medical management, including medicines and pulmonary rehabilitation, have been optimized. This includes maximizing therapy, while limiting steroids, through the hospitalization for the LVRS.[9] Patients need to be limited enough to justify LVRS, but not so debilitated that their risk for surgery is too high. Pulmonary plethysmography is important to make sure that the patient is in the right range to be considered for LVRS. Generally, appropriate surgical candidates have a forced expiratory volume in 1 second (FEV1) between 20% and 40% of predicted, TLC greater than 120%, a high RV (greater than 200%), and diffusing capacity for carbon monoxide (DLCO) between 20% and 40% of predicted. FEV1 or DLCO of less than 20% predicted have a higher risk of death.[10] The pulmonologist also helps with the perioperative management of these patients.

There are some developing roles for endobronchial valves in patients with emphysema, especially those with homogeneous emphysema, as LVRS increases mortality these patients.[3,7,11] It is often reserved for patients who have surgical contraindications or choose endobronchial valves.[1] An involved and expansive multidisciplinary team, including those interventional pulmonologists who place endobronchial valves, subsequently covers all plausible alternate therapies. Although emphysema has a spectrum of symptoms that occasionally will lead a patient down a path to pursue lung transplantation, it can be beneficial, but not required, to have pulmonologists involved in lung transplantation as members of the team.[8]

THORACIC SURGEON

The surgeon needs to be involved in the total management for LVRS. Although initially performed via sternotomy, safety and patient benefit via bilateral video-assisted thoracoscopic surgery has been demonstrated; therefore, a surgeon must be proficient in this technique.[12] Technical aspects, including the volume of lung removed and the buttressing of staple lines are critical to success.[13] A surgeon removing an insufficient volume of the upper lobe simply leads the patient to a forum of operative risk without potential benefit.[14] The surgeon needs to lead the team and understand all aspects of screening, selection, the operation, and postoperative care. Because emphysema can progress to lung transplantation, it can be beneficial, but not required, to have thoracic surgeons involved in lung transplantation as members of the LVRS multidisciplinary team.[8] The surgeon has the greatest to gain from a multidisciplinary team for treatment of LVRS. This surgery, as demonstrated by the NETT trial, carries much greater risk of complication and death in certain groups. The multidisciplinary team can help with this evaluation and risk stratification to ensure that patients receiving LVRS are the most ideal patients of success.

RADIOLOGIST

An understanding of the imaging of patients who are potential candidates is critical to a multidisciplinary group. Severely emphysematous lungs have good compliance so they expand well, but poor elastic recoil so they do not decompress well with expiration. The CT shows hyperexpanded lungs and flat diaphragms. The radiologic imaging is the most important most important criteria for LVRS. Ideal imaging should select nonfunctional areas of lung with poor elastic recoil to be resected and the opposite to remain. Unfortunately, no such imaging currently exists.

The CT scan is the most important imaging test to select candidates for LVRS. Thin-slice CT demonstrates the severity of emphysema better than the standard thicker (5-mm) slices of CT scans. The NETT used a scale of 1 to 4 grading of the amount of emphysema. The chest was divided into 4 sections and rated the amount of emphysema in cross sections in those 4 areas. Ratings were as follows: 1 (0%–25%), 2 (26%–50%), 3 (51%–75%), and 4 (76%–100%) as the % emphysema seen in cross sections. An example of significant heterogeneity would be 4 at the apex and 2 at the base.

The quantitative perfusion test is a good test to demonstrate heterogeneity. Most centers prefer to perform this at their center to avoid intertechnique variability.[1,8] Poor perfusion at the apex and good perfusion at the bases of the lungs documents good heterogeneity. There is occasional discordance between the quantitative perfusions scan and the CT scan.[8] Some centers will offer surgery to patients with heterogeneity localized to the lower lobes with appropriate patient counseling.[1] In some cases, the perfusion scan shows heterogeneity not seen on CT scan.

REHABILITATION COORDINATOR

Pulmonary rehabilitation is imperative for preoperative rehabilitation and patient selection for LVRS. Patients with severe emphysema are generally quite de-conditioned because their level of activity and exercise is severely limited. Per Medicare guidelines, patients for LVRS need to complete a pulmonary rehabilitation program before LVRS. This program spans 6 to 10 weeks.[9,15] This helps to recondition patients and reduce their complication rates postoperatively. A patient's exercise tolerance is assessed using a standard shuttle walk or a 6-minute walk test. After rehabilitation, patients are reassessed for surgical candidacy.[9] Another important benefit is that the rehabilitation coordinator can evaluate the patient's motivation.

The NETT demonstrated effectiveness of pulmonary rehabilitation and the centrality of its utilization to select appropriate candidates for surgery.[15] It was also initially designed to improve physical and psychological function, as well as educate patients on their own lung disease. These sessions involved supervised exercise, education, and psychosocial session by a mental health provider.[15] The use of pulmonary rehabilitation improved the 6-minute walk distance achieved, improvements in dyspnea, and quality of life.[15] Pulmonary rehabilitation produced substantial improvement in 20% of patients so they did not need LVRS.

In our experience, occasionally when we do a consultation for LVRS, patients will state that they are very motivated to move forward with an LVRS intervention and they want to be compliant with all instructions perioperatively and postoperatively. We had 2 such patients guarantee that they were highly motivated to succeed following the operation. Both awakened after their anesthetic to say they wanted to die. Aligning with their wish, they both did not comply with postoperative requirements and so, in fact, did die from pneumonia. Although patients may want to be compliant, pulmonary rehabilitation, under the direction of the coordinator, can ensure they have the will and strength to follow through. Sometimes the patients talk a good story but in reality, they are not motivated to achieve the outcomes required. Continuity and centralization of a coordinator running a program permits active involvement in rehabilitation as well as someone with insight and honesty on a patient's true level of motivation.

ANESTHESIOLOGIST

Although the anesthesiologist does not need to be an integral member of the selection team, the operative success of LVRS hinges on the appropriate management of these patients in the operating theater. The anesthesiologist must command a solid grasp of the pathophysiology of emphysema as well as the details of the LVRS itself.[16] Anesthesia should be proficient with one-lung ventilation and the use of epidural analgesia.[16] Patients will require standard lung isolation via a double lumen tube during the operation. For anesthesia, propofol is strongly considered, as it maintains pulmonary vasoconstriction decreasing the shunt fraction and does not rely on the lungs of elimination.[16] For intraoperative ventilation, it is key to realize that patients are at risk for barotrauma and gas trapping.[16] Pressure-controlled ventilation should be used rather than volume-controlled ventilation during the LVRS.[16] To avoid hyperinflation, a long inspiratory to expiratory ratio should be used (Q). It is also critical to monitor intraoperative carbon dioxide as patients undergo periods of single lung ventilation and this can limit gas exchange. Some level of hypercapnia will inevitably develop. Critical to success is early extubation, which should occur immediately after surgery to minimize the risks of the dreaded postoperative air leak.[16]

NURSING

To operate on patients with very poor pulmonary function can carry substantial risk. Our nurses had great pride of ownership that drove them to making sure patients did well. For example, 1 patient after LVRS had an arterial blood gas in the recovery room with a CO_2 of 140. The nurse caring for the patient did a fabulous job to make the patient breath better. The patient did not require reintubation and ultimately did very well. The goal was to not have any patients intubated in the recovery room or postoperatively in the hospital. Patients needed to ambulate 4 times a day in the hallways and actively participate in all aspects of pulmonary toilet postoperatively. Our overall results were very good because of the fine nursing care.

Table 1
Overlapping and different indications for LVRS and lung transplantation

Possible Indication	LVRS	Lung Transplantation
Heterogeneous	Yes	Yes
Homogeneous	No	Yes
Hyperinflated	Yes	No
Restricted	No	Yes
Emphysema	Yes	Yes
Fibrosis	No	Yes
Age, y	<75	<60

RESPIRATORY THERAPY

Chest physiotherapy is an important part to the postoperative recovery and should be used on postoperative day 1.[16] A center performing LVRS should have the appropriate patient support for respiratory therapy.

LUNG TRANSPLANTATION

Both LVRS and lung transplantation are reasonable treatments for selected patients with emphysema. The operations have some unique and some overlapping indications (**Table 1**). The LVRS team leaders need to understand both procedures to select the optimal treatment for patients with overlapping indications. The benefits from LVRS usually last a few years. Therefore, LVRS may be a better choice for a younger patient if lung transplantation is still an option after the benefit of LVRS is gone.

SUMMARY

Aside from the contribution to the team by different individuals, the multidisciplinary team must have guidelines on agreement of basic selection criteria, protocols, and assessments.[8] As mentioned previously, the provider who benefits the most from the multidisciplinary care team approach to LVRS is the surgeon. The person who supersedes this benefit is the patient, whether it is confirming their candidacy for LVRS or avoiding a poor outcome. As an inappropriate candidate for LVRS, the patient is set-up to be the greatest benefactor from and invested multidisciplinary team for LVRS. It cannot be reiterated enough that patient selection, as clearly outlined by the NETT, is the key to a successful LVRS program, so it is therefore inferred that the success of the program lies simply with those doing the selecting.

CLINICS CARE POINTS

- Identify highly motivated patients
- Avoid postoperative intubation
- Aggressive postoperative ambulation and pulmonary toilet
- Epidural catheters to facilitate postoperative pain control

---

DISCLOSURE

None.

REFERENCES

1. Rathinam S, Oey I, Steiner M, et al. The role of the emphysema multidisciplinary team in a successful lung volume reduction surgery programme†. Eur J Cardiothorac Surg 2014;46(6):1021–6.
2. Naunheim KS, Wood DE, Mohsenifar Z, et al. Long-term follow-up of patients receiving lung-volume-reduction surgery versus medical therapy for severe emphysema by the National Emphysema Treatment Trial Research Group. Ann Thorac Surg 2006;82(2):431–43.
3. Fishman A, Martinez F, Naunheim K, et al. A randomized trial comparing lung-volume-reduction surgery with medical therapy for severe emphysema. N Engl J Med 2003;348(21):2059–73.
4. McKenna RJ Jr, Brenner M, Fischel RJ, et al. Patient selection criteria for lung volume reduction surgery. J Thorac Cardiovasc Surg 1997;114(6): 957–67.
5. Brantigan OC, Mueller E. Surgical treatment of pulmonary emphysema. Am Surg 1957;23(9):789–804.
6. Cooper JD, Trulock EP, Triantafillou AN, et al. Bilateral pneumectomy (volume reduction) for chronic obstructive pulmonary disease. J Thorac Cardiovasc Surg 1995;109(1):106–19.
7. Marchetti N, Kaufman T, Chandra D, et al. Endobronchial coils versus lung volume reduction surgery or medical therapy for treatment of advanced homogenous emphysema. Chronic Obstr Pulm Dis 2018;5(2):87–96.
8. Oey I, Waller D. The role of the multidisciplinary emphysema team meeting in the provision of lung volume reduction. J Thorac Dis 2018;10(Suppl 23): S2824–9.
9. DeCamp MM Jr, Lipson D, Krasna M, et al. The evaluation and preparation of the patient for lung volume reduction surgery. Proc Am Thorac Soc 2008;5(4): 427–31.
10. National Emphysema Treatment Trial Research Group, Fishman A, Fessler H, et al. Patients at high risk of death after lung-volume-reduction surgery. N Engl J Med 2001;345(15):1075–83.
11. Gelb A, McKenna RJ Jr, Brenner M, et al. Contribution of lung and chest wall mechanics following emphysema resection. Chest 1996;110:11–7.
12. McKenna RJ Jr, Benditt JO, DeCamp M, et al. Safety and efficacy of median sternotomy versus video-assisted thoracic surgery for lung volume reduction surgery. J Thorac Cardiovasc Surg 2004;127(5): 1350–60.
13. Fischel RJ, McKenna RJ Jr. Bovine pericardium versus bovine collagen to buttress staples for lung reduction operations. Ann Thorac Surg 1998;65(1): 217–9.
14. Brenner M, McKenna RJ Jr, Chen JC, et al. Relationship between amount of lung resected and outcome after lung volume reduction surgery. Ann Thorac Surg 2000;69(2):388–93.
15. Ries AL, Make BJ, Lee SM, et al. The effects of pulmonary rehabilitation in the national emphysema treatment trial. Chest 2005;128(6):3799–809.
16. Hillier J, Gillbe C. Anaesthesia for lung volume reduction surgery. Anaesthesia 2003;58(12):1210–9.

Life Expectancy and Rate of Decline After Lung Volume Reduction Surgery

Sowmyanarayanan Thuppal, MD, PhD[a,b], Nicholas Lanzotti, MPH[a],
Bradley Vost, BS[a], Traves Crabtree, MD[a], Stephen Markwell, MA[a],
Benjamin Seadler, BS[a], Nisha Rizvi, PhD[a,b], Justin Sawyer, BS[a],
Kyle McCullough, MD[a], Stephen R. Hazelrigg, MD[a,*]

KEYWORDS

- Lung volume reduction surgery • Emphysema • Long-term outcomes • Survival rates
- Heterogeneous emphysema • Homogeneous emphysema

KEY POINTS

- Five-year survival rates post–lung volume reduction surgery (LVRS) for emphysema range between 63% and 78%.
- In well-selected patients with heterogeneous emphysema, there is a significant improvement in lung function at 5-years post-LVRS.
- There are durable improvements in disease-specific quality of life at 5 years post-LVRS.
- Select patients with homogenous emphysema may benefit from LVRS provided proper care is taken in resection of damaged tissue and careful patient selection.

INTRODUCTION

Chronic obstructive pulmonary disease (COPD), characterized by a spectrum of chronic bronchitis and emphysema, is one of the most debilitating lung conditions and is the fourth leading cause of death in the United States. Current treatment guidelines for COPD are focused on pulmonary rehabilitation and medical management with bronchodilators and inhaled corticosteroids, which have only been shown to decrease symptoms without prolonging patient survival.[1,2] Supplemental oxygen and smoking cessation are the only interventions shown to provide a survival benefit.[3,4] The high prevalence and mortality associated with COPD, along with limited treatment options, have spurred research into lung volume reduction surgery (LVRS) as a new treatment modality for advanced COPD.

LVRS was first described by Otto Brantigan in 1959.[5] He enrolled 57 patients with obstructive pulmonary emphysema over a period of 8 years. The procedure involved thoracotomy followed by unilateral removal of 20% to 30% of the diseased peripheral lung tissue in patients with emphysema. If the patient still was symptomatic, then the second side was operated on. Results of the study showed that 75% of the patients had symptomatic improvement but the early mortality rate was 16%. The procedure was not widely accepted largely due to difficulties in quantitating improvement and the early mortality rate of 16%. In 1983, Gaensler and colleagues[6] suggested that local resection should not be undertaken in patients with bullous emphysema.

Proper patient selection criteria were needed for performing lung volume reduction to improve the functional status and quality of life (QOL). Success

[a] Division of Cardiothoracic Surgery, Department of Surgery, SIU School of Medicine, 701 North 1st Street, Springfield, IL 62794-9679, USA; [b] Center for Clinical Research, SIU School of Medicine, 701 North 1st Street, Springfield, IL 62794-9679, USA
* Corresponding author.
E-mail address: shazelrigg@siumed.edu

Thorac Surg Clin 31 (2021) 177–188
https://doi.org/10.1016/j.thorsurg.2021.01.001
1547-4127/21/© 2021 Elsevier Inc. All rights reserved.

was reported and published in the early 1990s using thoracoscopic laser techniques. It was at times difficult to replicate these results and the LVRS techniques evolved to stapled resection of the hyperinflated diseased lung. In 1995, Cooper and colleagues[7] reported on LVRS and had performed the procedure in 20 patients without giant bullous emphysema but with very heterogeneous disease. The results showed promising improvement in lung function and QOL. Following this success, a larger study involving 150 patients with long-term follow-up was conducted.[8] All patients had severe dyspnea, increased lung capacity, hyperinflation, and heterogeneous disease. Bilateral LVRS was performed using a sternotomy with removal of 20% to 30% of the lung volume in each lung using a linear stapler and bovine pericardial strips for suture line buttressing. Most of the damaged tissue was removed from the upper lobe whereas 18 patients had lower lobe destruction warranting removal of damaged tissue. The results showed a significant increase in percentage predicted

value of forced expiratory volume in 1 second (FEV$_1$), a decrease in percentage predicted values of total lung capacity (TLC) and residual volume (RV), improved QOL with decreased oxygen, and corticosteroid use up to 2 years postsurgery. Following these studies, multiple studies were published that showed promising results with LVRS.

The current LVRS patient selection guidelines are based on the National Emphysema Treatment Trial (NETT),[9] a prospective clinical trial of 1218 subjects randomized to LVRS or medical treatment with a follow-up between 6 months and 4.5 years. The study enrolled patients with heterogenous and homogenous emphysema and predominantly upper lobe emphysema and non–upper lobe emphysema (including predominantly affecting the lower lobes, diffuse, or predominantly affecting the superior segments of the lower lobes). All enrolled subjects underwent 6 weeks to 10 weeks of pulmonary rehabilitation prior to randomization. The study concluded that patients

Table 1
Baseline demographic characteristics, functional and clinical outcomes in patients with emphysema undergoing lung volume reduction surgery by upper lobe perfusion

Characteristics	Upper Lobe Perfusion Less than or Equal to 15% (n = 66)	Upper Lobe Perfusion Greater than 15% (n = 69)
Age, years, mean (SD)	66.4 (±7.6)	66.6 (±7.6)
BMI, kg/m^2, mean (SD)	24.9 (±4.4)	25.2 (±4.6)
Gender (female)	34 (52%)	25 (36%)
Race/ethnicity		
Non-Hispanic white	64 (98%)	66 (96%)
Non-Hispanic black	1 (2%)	3 (4%)
Smoking history		
10–19 pack-years	0 (0%)	1 (1%)
20–29 pack-years	1 (2%)	6 (9%)
30–39 pack-years	10 (15%)	6 (9%)
40–49 pack-years	8 (12%)	7 (10%)
50–59 pack-years	5 (8%)	8 (12%)
60+ pack-years	42 (64%)	39 (58%)
FVC, % predicted value	66 (53–75)	67 (52–84)
FEV$_1$, % predicted value	25 (22–30.5)	24.5 (21–32.3)
RV, % predicted value	215 (192–267)	216 (190–240.5)
DLCO, % predicted value	38 (28–45)	37.5 (31.3–46.8)
6MWD (ft)	1194 (1030–1400)	1200 (1038–1350)
Paco$_2$ (mm Hg)	42 (38–63)	41 (35.8–44.7)
Pao$_2$ (mm Hg)	69 (63–74)	68 (61–71.2)

Abbreviations: BMI, body mass index; DLCO, diffusing capacity for carbon monoxide; FEV1, forced expiratory volume in the first second; FVC, forced vital capacity; PaCO2, partial pressure of carbon dioxide; PaO2, partial pressure of oxygen; RV, residual volume; 6MWD, 6 minute walk distance test.

with both predominantly upper lobe emphysema and low baseline exercise capacity had a survival advantage. Because of the increased mortality and poor improvement in functional outcomes, patients with non–upper lobe emphysema and low baseline exercise capacity were determined as poor candidates for LVRS. Several studies with similar inclusion criteria have shown that LVRS is effective during the short-term follow-up when well selected; however, few studies have looked at long-term outcomes post-LVRS in patients with end-stage emphysema. This review looks at studies that followed-up patients for at least 24 months from the time of surgery.

HETEROGENOUS EMPHYSEMA

The NETT trial recommended LVRS for patients with predominantly upper lobe emphysema with low exercise capacity. At 24 months' follow-up, the risk of death in patients with emphysema with predominantly upper lobe emphysema with low exercise capacity undergoing LVRS was 0.47 and there was an improvement in maximum workload (W) by more than 10-W, with improvement in St. George's Respiratory Questionnaire Scores.[9] At 5 years, the risk of death was 0.67 with improvement of St. George's Respiratory Questionnaire Scores. The improvement in workload, however, was durable only up to 3 years.[10] Long-term follow-up of NETT patients showed the mortality rates in LVRS patients was significantly lower (0.11 deaths per person-year) compared with the medical group (0.13 deaths per person-year), in spite of increased early mortality in the LVRS group.[10] At 5-year follow-up, there was a sustained improvement in lung function indicators, including FEV_1 (+1.4%), forced vital capacity

Table 2
Relative change from baseline (% change) in clinical and functional outcomes in patients with emphysema undergoing lung volume reduction surgery over 5-year period by upper lobe perfusion status

Outcomes	Upper Lobe Perfusion Less than or Equal to 15%, median (interquartile range)		
	Year 1 (n = 43)	Year 3 (n = 27)	Year 5 (n = 15)
FVC, % predicted value	41.4 (23.5–62.1)[c]	28.6 (20.0–45.2)[c]	21.2 (−4.2–36.1)[a]
FEV_1, % predicted value	54.2 (26.3–72.7)[c]	22.7 (12.0–51.5)[c]	22.2 (−10.0–37.5)[a]
RV, % predicted value	−27.8 (−42.5 to −18.3)[c]	−21.9 (−30.3 to −13.6)[c]	−12.1 (−23.8 to −2.6)[a]
DLCO, % predicted value	16.2 (0.0–28.2)[c]	12.3 (−5.8–25.6)[a]	8.7 (−13.3–26.2)
6MWD (ft)	9.3 (2.2–20.0)[c]	1.4 (−5.4–16.1)	−0.6 (−29.2–9.1)
$Paco_2$ (mm Hg)	−5.3 (−16.7–2.6)[a]	2.2 (−6.3–7.0)	2.3 (−10.7–9.8)
Pao_2 (mm Hg)	7.7 (0.0–20.9)[b]	1.4 (−11.3–25.2)	2.9 (−1.8–10.8)
Outcomes	Upper Lobe Perfusion greater than15%		
	Year 1 (n = 31)	Year 3 (n = 22)	Year 5 (n = 12)
FVC, % predicted value	27.7 (11.1–71.4)[c]	21.0 (2.9 45.2)[b]	30.8 (12.8–74.2)[a]
FEV_1, % predicted value	23.8 (6.2–56.0)[c]	23.7 (−5.1–34.2)[a]	37.5 (6.6–61.4)[a]
RV, % predicted value	−16.8 (−32.6 to −6.93)[c]	−14.6 (−21.9–3.5)	−1.6 (−20.5–2.6)
DLCO, % predicted value	7.3 (−2.4–17.8)[a]	−4.3 (−17.2–20.0)	−2.1 (−13.9–20.3)
6MWD (ft)	2.8 (−4.9–16.3)	−12.2 (−28.1–9.1)	−2.0 (−16.5–7.3)
$Paco_2$ (mm Hg)	−4.5 (−9.8–7.5)	5.0 (−3.3–9.8)	5.6 (−12.5–20.5)
Pao_2 (mm Hg)	0.0 (−2.9–14.5)	1.5 (−5.9–14.7)	1.3 (−10.6–27.3)

Abbreviations: DLCO, diffusing capacity for carbon monoxide; FEV1, forced expiratory volume in the first second; FVC, forced vital capacity; PaCO2, partial pressure of carbon dioxide; PaO2, partial pressure of oxygen; RV, residual volume; 6MWD, 6 minute walk distance test.
[a] $P<.05$.
[b] $P<.001$.
[c] $P<.0001$.

Table 3
Quality of life utility scores—baseline and change from baseline at 1 year, 3 years, and 5 years in patients with emphysema undergoing lung volume reduction surgery by upper lobe perfusion status—

	Upper Lobe Perfusion Less than or Equal to 15%, median (interquartile range)				Upper Lobe Perfusion Greater than 15%, median (interquartile range)			
	Baseline	Change at year 1 (n = 41)	Change at year 3 (n = 37)	Change at year 5 (n = 22)	Baseline	Change at year 1 (n = 33)	Change at year 3 (n = 22)	Change at year 5 (n = 17)
EQ-5D	0.71 (0.52–0.85)	0.07 (0.03–0.21)[c]	0.04 (−0.07–0.14)	−0.00 (−0.12–0.07)	0.74 (0.60–0.81)	0.70 (0–0.12)[a]	0.00 (−0.10–0.04)	0.00 (−0.12–0.10)
SF-36								
General health	35 (30–55)	20 (0–25)[c]	0 (−10–20)	5 (−15–15)	40 (25–50)	10 (0–15)[a]	−5 (−15–0)	−6.2 (−15–0)
Physical functioning	23 (10–30)	35 (20–40)[c]	20 (5–35)[c]	2.5 (−10–35)	18 (8.8–31)	25 (5–45)[c]	5 (0–15)[a]	20 (−5–30.7)[a]
Energy/fatigue	42.5 (30–55)	25 (10–45)[c]	10 (0–30)[c]	10 (−10–20)	47.5 (33.8–55)	10 (−10–30)[a]	0 (−10–20)	0 (−5–15)
Bodily pain	90 (77.5–100)	0 (0–10)	0 (−22.5–0)	0 (−20–0)	100 (79.4–100)	0 (−20–10)	0 (0–10)	0 (−25–0)
Emotional well-being	72 (61–88)	8 (0–20)[a]	8 (−4–12)[a]	0 (−12–8)	74 (60–90.6)	0 (−4–8)	−4 (−20–4)	0 (−4–4)
Social functioning	75 (50–87.5)	12.5 (0–37.5)[b]	12.5 (−12.5–25)	−6.2 (−37.5–12.5)	75 (50–90.6)	0 (−12.5–25)	0 (−12.5–25)	0 (−12.5–37.5)
Role limitations due to physical health	0 (0–25)	50 (25–100)[c]	0 (0–75)[a]	12.5 (0–50)[a]	0 (0–50)	25 (0–50)[c]	0 (−25–25)	0 (−25–25)
Role limitations due to emotional problems	83.3 (33.3–100)	0 (0–33.3)	0 (−33.3–0)	0 (−33.3–0)	100 (33.3–100)	0 (0–0)	0 (−66.7–0)[a]	0 (−33.3–0)[a]

[a] P<.05.
[b] P<.001.
[c] P<.0001.

(FVC) (+3.44%), and RV (−19.49%) of the predicted values. There was an overall 0.89-W improvement in maximum workload, −4.12 improvement in shortness of breath score, and 0.088 improvement in quality of well-being scores.[11] Based on the results from NETT study, LVRS was found to have a long-term durable effect on patients with emphysema with improvement in both functional and physiologic outcomes.

The authors followed 66 patients with predominantly upper lobe emphysema (ventilation-perfusion ratio [V/Q] ≤15%) for up to 5 years. Mean age was 66 years old, and 64% of the patients had a smoking history of 60 or more pack-years. All patients underwent 20 supervised pulmonary rehabilitation sessions prior to LVRS. Baseline mean values were FEV_1, 25% of predicted value; FVC, 66% of predicted value; RV, 215% of predicted value; and diffusing capacity of the lungs for carbon monoxide (DLCO), 38% of predicted value. The 6-minute walk distance (6MWD) was 1194 ft at baseline. Arterial oxygen and carbon dioxide were 42 mm Hg and 69 mm Hg, respectively (**Table 1**). At 5-year follow-up, there remained a significant improvement in FEV_1 (22%), FVC (22%), and RV (−12%) compared with baseline (**Table 2**). Improvement in DLCO was durable at 3 years whereas arterial pressure of oxygen and carbon dioxide was durable only up to 1 year follow-up (see **Table 2**). Based on the 36-item Short Form Health Survey (SF-36) QOL questionnaire, physical functioning, energy, and emotional well-being improved significantly compared with baseline and was durable up to 3 years post-LVRS. The limitation due to physical health, however, was significantly less compared with baseline values at 5-years post-LVRS (**Table 3**). Survival rates at 1 year, 2 years, 3 years, 4 years, and 5 years were 92.4%, 90.7%, 85.4%, 79%, and 69%, respectively (**Fig. 1**). The numbers of deaths at 1 year, 3 years, and 5 years post-LVRS in this group were 5 patients, 4 patients, and 7 patients. At the end of 5 years, 23 patients were lost to follow-up; however, there was no difference in baseline demographic and functional outcomes between those who did and did not complete 5-years of follow-up.

Five-year survival rates in patients undergoing LVRS for heterogeneous emphysema range between 63% and 78% (**Table 4**).[12–18] There was a significant improvement in overall QOL, measured using EuroQol-5D (EQ-5D) and SF-36 questionnaires up to 1 years to 3 years post-LVRS; however, studies have shown improvement in disease specific modified Medical Research Council scale and St. George's Respiratory Questionnaire up to 5-years post-LVRS.[10,12,13,15] The 6MWD improved significantly beyond year 1 and was durable up to 5-years.[14,19] There is a significant improvement in lung function up to 5-years of follow-up post-LVRS.[11,13,14] In well-selected patients with heterogeneous emphysema, LVRS has a durable long-term outcome up to 5-years of follow-up.

HOMOGENOUS EMPHYSEMA

It is postulated that improvements in lung function post-LVRS are due to reduction in RV and functional RV, leading to increased elastic recoil, thereby reducing airflow obstruction and hyperinflation. These benefits do not depend on lung morphology and hence improvement post-LVRS should be measurable not only in patients with heterogeneous emphysema but also in select patients with homogeneous emphysema. In patients with homogeneous emphysema, however, resection of damaged tissue may involve removal of some healthy parenchyma, leading to compensatory hyperinflation.

In the NETT study, 69 patients who had FEV_1 less than 20% of the predicted value with either homogeneous emphysema on CT or DLCO of less than 20% of their predicted value were considered a very-high-risk group. The 30-day mortality in these patients was 16% and hence the data monitoring board stopped recruiting these high-risk patients. Based on the results from already enrolled patients, there was minimal improvement in 6MWD and FEV_1, percentage of predicted value, at 6 months with no improvement in QOL.[20]

Weder and colleagues,[21] in 1997, published post-LVRS outcomes in 17 patients (mean age of 66 years) with homogeneous emphysema, with a baseline FEV_1 of 27% of predicted value, FVC 66% of predicted value, and RV 251% of predicted value. At 3-months' follow-up there were significant improvements in FEV_1, FVC, and RV. There also was significant improvement in arterial O_2 content and decline in CO_2 content. There was no mortality among these patients (**Table 5**).

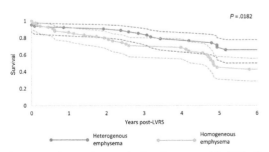

Fig. 1. Kaplan-Meier survival estimates, with 95% CI, by type of emphysema.

Table 4
Inclusion criteria and outcomes post–lung volume reduction surgery in patients with heterogeneous emphysema

Study	Mean Age, Years	Heterogeneous Emphysema Diagnosis	Outcomes Time Points	Forced Expiratory Volume in the First Second of Expiration, Percentage of Predicted Value	Forced Vital Capacity, Percentage of Predicted Value	Residual Volume, Percentage of Predicted Value	Diffusing Capacity of the Lungs for Carbon Monoxide, Percentage of Predicted Value	Six-minute Walk Distance, Feet	Quality of Life	Survival (%)
Yusen et al,[15] 2003	61	Computed tomography	Baseline (n = 200) 12 mo (n = 185) 36 mo (n = 139) 60 mo (n = 33)	25		282	29	345 meters	mMRC 2.4 – 1.9 2.1	Survival 93 83 63
Horwood et al,[18] 2019	63	Computed tomography	Baseline (n = 135) 24 mo (n = 69) 60 mo (n = 31)	29	75	218	35.5	807		Survival 91 71
Ginsburg et al,[17] 2016	62.5		Baseline (n = 91) 24 mo (n = 41) 60 mo (n = 18)							Survival 97 79
Agzarian et al,[16] 2013	64		Baseline (n = 32)	25		5.4 L	31	340 meters		Survival 48 mo - 56 72 mo - 42 96 mo - 37
Ciccone et al,[14] 2003	62	Computed tomography	Baseline (n = 249) 12 mo (n = 225) 36 mo (n = 178) 60 mo (n = 106)	26 38 34 30		277 193 198 222	33 39 36 34	1142 1341 1271 1154		Survival 93 84 67
Fujimoto et al,[13] 2002			Baseline (n = 88) 12 mo (n = 57) 24 mo (n = 46) 36 mo (n = 26) 60 mo	27.5 31.1 30.3 30.1				285 m 390 m 349 m 334 m	mMRC 1.5 2.0 2.1	Survival 83 71
Hamacher et al,[12] 1999	66	Computed tomography	Baseline (n = 18) 24 mo (n = 18)	31 41		217 172		252 m 352 m	mMRC 3.4 3.4 1.9	

Weder et al,[19] 2009	64	Computed tomography and lung perfusion scintigraphy	Baseline (n = 112)	29	38.8	797	Survival
			12 mo (n = 70)	39	43	1263	96
			24 mo (n = 58)	38	43	1233	93
			36 mo (n = 38)	33	41	1266	77
			60 mo (n = 27)	33	38.7	1207	40

All follow-up values presented in the table are significant compared with baseline value.

Table 5
Inclusion criteria and outcomes post–lung volume reduction surgery in patients with homogeneous emphysema

Study	Inclusion/ Exclusion Criteria	Mean Age, Years	Homogeneous Emphysema Diagnosis	Outcomes Time Points	Forced Expiratory Volume in the First Second of Expiration, Percentage of Predicted Value	Forced Vital Capacity, Percentage of Predicted Value	Residual Volume, Percentage of Predicted Value	Diffusing Capacity of the Lungs for Carbon Monoxide, Percentage of Predicted Value	Six-minute Walk Distance, Feet	Quality of Life	Survival (%)
Weder et al,[19] 2009	Inclusion: FEV$_1$ <40% predicted value TLC >120% predicted value mMRC ≥ grade 2 Exclusion: FEV$_1$ <20% predicted value and DLCO <20% predicted value and advanced parenchymal destruction	64	Computed tomography and lung perfusion scintigraphy	Baseline (n=138) 12 mo (n = 78) 24 mo (n = 57) 36 mo (n = 37) 60 mo (n = 21)	28 35 36	75 87 91		39.9 43 45	807 1141 1119	mMRC 3.46 1.7 2.1	Survival 96 88 70 48

Study	Inclusion/Exclusion	Imaging	Age	Timepoints						
Bloch et al,[22] 2002	Inclusion: FEV$_1$ <40% predicted value, RV >200% predicted value; Exclusion: DLCO <20% predicted value	Computed tomography		Baseline (n=27), 12 mo (n = 20), 24 mo (n = 16)	25, 35, 31					
NETT Research Group, 2001,[20] and Kaplan et al,[24] 2014	NETT selection criteria	Computed tomography	63	Baseline (n=70), 30-d (n = 58), 52 mo	17.1	267.4	20.5	1038	Quality of well-being scale, 0.58	mortality 16%
Hamacher et al,[12] 1999	—	Computed tomography	66	Baseline (n=12), 3 mo, 24 mo	26, 38, 32	234, 193, 203		274, meters	mMRC 3.5, 1.6, 2.0	
Weder et al,[21] 1997	Inclusion: FEV$_1$ <1.2 L, TLC >130% predicted value; Exclusion: Paco$_2$ >55 mm Hg, DLCO <201%	Computed tomography	62	Baseline (n=17), 3 mo (n = 17)	27, ~36.9	251	66	249, meters	mMRC 3.6	

Abbreviations: DLCO, diffusing capacity for carbon monoxide; FEV1, forced expiratory volume in the first second; mMRC, modified medical research council scale; NETT, national emphysema treatment trial; PaCO2, partial pressure of carbon dioxide; RV, residual volume; TLC, total lung capacity.
All follow-up values presented in the table are significant compared with baseline value.

Hamacher and colleagues,[12] in 1999, performed LVRS in 12 patients with homogeneous emphysema with a mean age of 66 years. Baseline FEV_1 was 26% of predicted value and RV was 234% of predicted value. Both FEV_1 and RV significantly improved at 3-months and 2 years post-LVRS, with increase in arterial O_2 and decrease in CO_2. Survival rate at 2-years was approximately 50%. Bloch and colleagues,[22] in 2002, also showed that there was a significant improvement in functional outcomes at 2-years post-LVRS in 27 patients with homogeneous emphysema with a baseline FEV_1 of 25% of predicted value and FVC of 79% of predicted value. The first study with a larger sample size, of 138 patients, with homogeneous emphysema was conducted by Weder and colleagues,[23] in 2009. Baseline FEV_1 was 28% of predicted value, FVC was 75% of predicted value, DLCO was 40% of predicted value, and 6MWD was 807 ft. All values improved significantly over the first 2 years post-LVRS. The values were still above the baseline value at 5 years, even though there was a lack of statistical significance probably due to a very small number of patients (n = 21) at 5-year follow-up. Survival rate was 96% at year 1, 70% at year 3, and 48% at year 5 of follow-up.

After a careful review of the literature, the authors performed LVRS in 69 patients categorized as homogeneous emphysema based on V/Q. All patients underwent 20 supervised sessions of cardiopulmonary rehabilitation. If the V/Q for the upper lobe was greater than 15%, then they were considered as having homogeneous emphysema. The median FEV_1 percentage of predicted value was 24.5 (interquartile ratio [IQR]: 21–32.3), DLCO of 37.5% of the predicted value (IQR: 31.3–46.8), FVC percentage predicted value of 67% (IQR: 52–84), RV was 216 of percentage of predicted value, and 6MWD was 1200 ft (see **Table 2**). Mean age of the sample was 66 years and approximately 60% of them had a smoking history of 60 or more pack-years. All baseline demographic, functional, and clinical outcomes were similar to those of patients undergoing LVRS with heterogeneous emphysema (V/Q ≤15%).

At the end of 1 year, both FEV_1 percentage of predicted value and FVC percentage of predicted value improved compared with baseline and the improvement lasted for up to 5 years post-LVRS (see **Table 3**); although RV and DLCO improved at first 2 years, the improvement was not durable beyond year 2. QOL improved during year 1 based on EQ-5D questionnaire, but there was no improvement beyond year 1. Similar results were seen with the general health

component of the SF-36 questionnaire. The physical functioning component of SF-36 questionnaire, however, significantly improved from baseline up to 5 years of follow-up. There were 9 deaths, 9 deaths, and 12 deaths at years 1 year, 3 years, and 5 years, respectively. At year 1, 2 patients sent the QOL questionnaire by mail and could not come for testing for lung functions; likewise, 5 patients sent in their QOL questionnaire but did not come for measuring functional outcomes at year 5. At the end of 5 years, 16 patients were lost to follow-up; however, there were no significant differences in baseline and functional outcomes between patients who did and did not complete 5 years of follow-up. There was a steady decline in survival percentage from 87% at year 1 to 71% at year 3 and 45% at year 5 (**Fig. 1**).

Based on the results from Weder and colleagues[23] and from the authors' center, select patients with homogeneous emphysema might benefit from LVRS with improved survival, functional, and QOL outcomes. Patients with homogeneous emphysema with baseline FEV_1 greater than 20% of predicted value and DLCO greater than 20% of predicted value may have better outcomes with LVRS provided proper care is taken in resection of damaged tissue with minimal removal of healthy parenchyma, thereby preventing compensatory hyperinflation. Future studies with larger sample size, improved selection of patients, appropriate resection of damaged tissue, and long-term follow-up will help in identifying eligible patients with homogeneous emphysema for LVRS.

SUMMARY

Most of the survival data pertain to heterogeneous disease. It seems that typically the improvement from LVRS with regard to pulmonary function tests is sustained for 3 years to 5 years. Five-year survival rates range from 63% to 78%. It would be expect patients follow expected survival in a similar medically treated population after that point.

The maturation of the VATS approach since the publication of the NETT trial, coupled with increased experience with LVRS at high-volume centers, has acted both to continuously improve long-term outcomes and to decrease surgical mortality. Data from the authors' study, coupled with recently published data from other centers, further bolster the broader usage of LVRS in patients appropriately selected for the surgery with end-stage emphysema. More importance should be given in selection of patients, as described by the NETT study; however, some select patients with homogeneous emphysema with hyperinflation may benefit from LVRS. Due to the unavailability of long-term data, the number of LVRSs performed have declined over the years. Based on the available data, LVRS seems a durable alternative for end-stage emphysema in patients not eligible for lung transplantation.

CLINICS CARE POINTS

- Five-year survival post-LVRS ranges from 63% to 78%.
- There are durable improvements in QOL, even at 5 years post-LVRS.
- Some carefully selected homogeneously distributed emphysema patients can benefit from LVRS.
- LVRS is a durable and effective option for patients with heterogeneous disease. It probably is underutilized.

DISCLOSURE

The authors have nothing to disclose.

REFERENCE

1. Calverley PM, Anderson JA, Celli B, et al. Salmeterol and fluticasone propionate and survival in chronic obstructive pulmonary disease. N Engl J Med 2007;356(8):775–89.
2. Salpeter SR. Bronchodilators in COPD: impact of beta-agonists and anticholinergics on severe exacerbations and mortality. Int J Chron Obstruct Pulmon Dis 2007;2(1):11–8.
3. Bai J-W, Chen X-X, Liu S, et al. Smoking cessation affects the natural history of COPD. Int J Chron Obstruct Pulmon Dis 2017;12:3323–8.
4. Pavlov N, Haynes AG, Stucki A, et al. Long-term oxygen therapy in COPD patients: population-based cohort study on mortality. Int J Chron Obstruct Pulmon Dis 2018;13:979–88.
5. Brantigan OC, Mueller E, Kress MB. A surgical approach to pulmonary emphysema. Am Rev Respir Dis 1959;80(1, Part 2):194–206.
6. Gaensler EA, Cugell DW, Knudson RJ, et al. Surgical management of emphysema. Clin Chest Med 1983;4(3):443–63.
7. Cooper JD, Trulock EP, Triantafillou AN, et al. Bilateral pneumectomy (volume reduction) for chronic obstructive pulmonary disease. J Thorac Cardiovasc Surg 1995;109(1):106–16 [discussion 116–09].
8. Cooper JD, Patterson GA, Sundaresan RS, et al. Results of 150 consecutive bilateral lung volume reduction procedures in patients with severe emphysema. J Thorac Cardiovasc Surg 1996;112(5):1319–29 [discussion 1329–30].
9. Fishman A, Martinez F, Naunheim K, et al. A randomized trial comparing lung-volume-reduction surgery with medical therapy for severe emphysema. N Engl J Med 2003;348(21):2059–73.
10. Naunheim KS, Wood DE, Mohsenifar Z, et al. Long-term follow-up of patients receiving lung-volume-reduction surgery versus medical therapy for severe emphysema by the National emphysema treatment trial research group. Ann Thorac Surg 2006;82(2):431–43.
11. Lim E, Sousa I, Shah PL, et al. Lung volume reduction surgery: reinterpreted with longitudinal data analyses methodology. Ann Thorac Surg 2020;109(5):1496–501.
12. Hamacher J, Bloch KE, Stammberger U, et al. Two years' outcome of lung volume reduction surgery in different morphologic emphysema types. Ann Thorac Surg 1999;68(5):1792–8.
13. Fujimoto T, Teschler H, Hillejan L, et al. Long-term results of lung volume reduction surgery. Eur J Cardiothorac Surg 2002;21(3):483–8.
14. Ciccone AM, Meyers BF, Guthrie TJ, et al. Long-term outcome of bilateral lung volume reduction in 250 consecutive patients with emphysema. J Thorac Cardiovasc Surg 2003;125(3):513–25.
15. Yusen RD, Lefrak SS, Gierada DS, et al. A prospective evaluation of lung volume reduction surgery in 200 consecutive patients. Chest 2003;123(4):1026–37.
16. Agzarian J, Miller JD, Kosa SD, et al. Long-term survival analysis of the Canadian lung volume reduction surgery trial. Ann Thorac Surg 2013;96(4):1217–22.
17. Ginsburg ME, Thomashow BM, Bulman WA, et al. The safety, efficacy, and durability of lung-volume reduction surgery: a 10-year experience. J Thorac Cardiovasc Surg 2016;151(3):717–24.e711.
18. Horwood CR, Mansour D, Abdel-Rasoul M, et al. Long-term results after lung volume reduction surgery: a single institution's experience. Ann Thorac Surg 2019;107(4):1068–73.
19. Weder W, Tutic M, Bloch KE. Lung volume reduction surgery in nonheterogeneous emphysema. Thorac Surg Clin 2009;19(2):193–9.
20. National Emphysema Treatment Trial Research G, Fishman A, Fessler H, et al. Patients at high risk of death after lung-volume-reduction surgery. N Engl J Med 2001;345(15):1075–83.
21. Weder W, Thurnheer R, Stammberger U, et al. Radiologic emphysema morphology is associated with outcome after surgical lung volume reduction. Ann Thorac Surg 1997;64(2):313–9 [discussion 319–20].

22. Bloch KE, Georgescu CL, Russi EW, et al. Gain and subsequent loss of lung function after lung volume reduction surgery in cases of severe emphysema with different morphologic patterns. J Thorac Cardiovasc Surg 2002;123(5):845–54.

23. Weder W, Tutic M, Lardinois D, et al. Persistent benefit from lung volume reduction surgery in patients with homogeneous emphysema. Ann Thorac Surg 2009;87(1):229–36 [discussion 236–27].

24. Kaplan RM, Sun Q, Naunheim KS, et al. Long-term follow-up of high-risk patients in the National Emphysema Treatment Trial. Ann Thorac Surg 2014;98: 1782–9.

Bronchoscopic Valve Treatment of End-Stage Chronic Obstructive Pulmonary Disease

Traves D. Crabtree, MD

KEYWORDS

- Endobronchial valve • Chronic obstructive pulmonary disease (COPD)
- Lung volume reduction surgery

KEY POINTS

- With appropriate patient selection, endobronchial valve therapy provides clinical improvement in forced volume of expiration in 1 second (FEV_1), walk distance, and quality of life in patients with end-stage chronic obstructive lung disease.
- Complications with endobronchial valve treatment are less than those historically been reported for lung volume reduction surgery.
- Post-treatment pneumothorax can be a significant complication after endobronchial valve therapy and may occur early or have a delayed presentation.

INTRODUCTION

Emphysema continues to be a significant cause of morbidity and mortality in the United States and worldwide. Despite optimal medical management, survivors with end-stage emphysema are significantly limited in their functional status, with associated poor patient-reported outcomes and quality of life.[1] It is in this subset of patients where surgical and endoscopic interventions hope to improve survival, quality of life, and functional capacity.

Irreversible destruction of alveolar tissue results in increased size of air spaces distal to the terminal bronchioles. This destruction and coalescence of alveoli lead to loss of elastic recoil within the lung tissue that causes small airways to collapse, leading to a functional obstruction of gas outflow with subsequent air trapping and dynamic hyperinflation of the lungs. Over time, this process results in lung and chest wall hyperexpansion, limiting inspiratory capacity and increasing work of breathing.

Surgical or interventional treatments attempt to resect or functionally limit flow to disproportionately hyperexpanded portions of the lung in an effort to redistribute ventilation to healthier lung tissue with better perfusion. Surgical removal of hyperexpanded portions of lung, or lung volume reduction surgery (LVRS), has a long history but was reinvigorated in the current era with the work of Dr Joel Cooper.[2] As outlined in previous articles, the National Emphysema Treatment Trial (NETT) demonstrated a significant improvement in survival with bilateral LVRS in addition to improvements in FEV_1, 6-minute walk distance (6MWD), quality of life, and dyspnea scores in well-selected patients with severe emphysema.[3,4] Using appropriate selection criteria in patients with heterogeneous disease, 90-day mortality was 5.2% (vs 1.5% in medically treated control group).[3,4] Despite the demonstration of the clinical efficacy of LVRS in the NETT trial, utilization of LVRS for the treatment of severe symptomatic emphysema has been disappointingly limited.

Division of Cardiothoracic Surgery, Department of Surgery, Southern Illinois University School of Medicine, 701 N. First Street D252, Springfield, IL 62794-9679, USA
E-mail address: Tcrabtree53@siumed.edu

Thorac Surg Clin 31 (2021) 189–201
https://doi.org/10.1016/j.thorsurg.2021.01.002
1547-4127/21/Published by Elsevier Inc.

This is multifactorial but partially related to a reticence to refer patients for LVRS because of the surgery-related morbidity and mortality.[5] This concern was the impetus to identify less invasive techniques that mimic the physiologic impact of LVRS.

Endobronchial valves (EBVs) were developed to block inspiration of air into severely diseased pulmonary segments while allowing egress of air to produce atelectasis of the target segment or lobe (**Fig. 1**). Multiple valves are available commercially and generally comprise a metal matrix covered in silicone. The valves come in different diameters and lengths to accommodate various sizes of segmental bronchi. The valves easily are deployed via standard flexible bronchoscopy either under general anesthesia or monitored sedation.

INDICATIONS

Indications for utilization of EBVs have evolved since their inception, but there still is significant overlap with indications for traditional surgical LVRS. General indications, with some variability based on the trial, include FEV_1 less than 45% to 50% predicted and greater than 15% to 20% predicted, hyperinflation with total lung capacity greater than 100%, residual volume (RV) greater than 150% predicted, limited exercise capacity (ie, 6MWD <450 m), and dyspnea (ie, Medical Research Council [MRC] dyspnea score >3), in patients undergoing optimal medical therapy. Patients also are required to quit smoking and to participate in pulmonary rehabilitation. Most trials have been limited to patients with smoking-related disease, although additional series have suggested a benefit in patients with α_1-antitrypsin deficiency.[6,7]

Initial studies of EBV therapy, as with LVRS, generally focused on patients with heterogeneous predominantly upper lobe disease. Subsequent series have suggested that EBV therapy may be beneficial in select patients with homogeneous

disease.[8] Relative exclusion criteria include severe coexisting comorbidity restricting exercise capacity or having an impact on overall survival, significant daily sputum production, giant bullae, pulmonary hypertension, or patients considered too frail to undergo complex bronchoscopic procedures.

ASSESSMENT OF COLLATERAL VENTILATION

Essential criteria include selection of patients with limited collateral ventilation to the target lobe. Objective assessment of collateral ventilation can be performed utilizing high-resolution computed tomography (HRCT) evaluation of fissure completeness (ideally >90%).[9] HRCT also is utilized to identify the ideal target lobe with the greatest degree of emphysema destruction based on Hounsfield units and to assess the degree of heterogeneity (>10%–15% difference vs ipsilateral lobe). Software has been developed to help standardize the initial HRCT assessment of fissure completeness and the severity of emphysematous destruction and is essential for the planning and work-up of these patients.

More contemporary trials have supplemented the HRCT assessment with utilization of the Chartis system (Pulmonx, Redwood City, California) to establish formal objective assessment of collateral ventilation. Using bronchoscopic-guided balloon catheter occlusion with a central channel, the Chartis system can measure air flow from the occluded segment/lobe. With the Chartis output graph, demonstration of continuous expiratory flow indicates collateral ventilation whereas a flow curve declining to zero indicates no collateral ventilation.[10]

Other studies have solely utilized HRCT, rather than supplementing with Chartis, to visually estimate the completeness of fissures. These reports suggest that HRCT and Chartis alone may be similar in accuracy (75%–84%) for classification of collateral ventilation and that HRCT may decrease procedure time and procedure-related costs for target lobe assessment during valve deployment.[10–12] The combined use of HRCT plus Chartis has a reported accuracy of 90% and allows evaluation of a broader range of patients with fissure scores as low as 80%. Pulmonary scintigraphy also is performed routinely to objectively quantify the degree of perfusion and aid in the selection of the target lobe.

PREDEFINED OUTCOME MEASURES

Most clinical trials have utilized outcome variables previously used in the evaluation of LVRS, including changes in pulmonary function tests

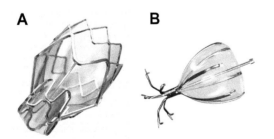

A   **B**

Fig. 1. (*A*) Pulmonx EBV. (*B*) Spiration Valve System (SVS). (*Courtesy of* Pulmonx Corp, Redwood City, California, with permission; and Olympus, Center Valley, PA, with permission.)

(ie, FEV$_1$), exercise capacity, and quality of life assessment. Efforts also have been made to standardize what would be considered the minimal clinically important difference (MCID) for assessment of change in chronic obstructive pulmonary disease (COPD) treatment strategies. Suggested criteria for MCID include at least a 10% increase in FEV$_1$ from baseline, at least a 26-m increase in 6MWD, and at least a 0.4-point improvement in the St. George's Respiratory Questionnaire (SGRQ).[13–15]

EARLY CLINICAL RESULTS

Table 1 provides a summary of outcomes associated with clinical trials of EBV therapy in patients with severe end-stage emphysema. Early trials of EBV therapy attempted to focus on bilateral partial occlusion of upper lobe predominant disease similar to the physiologic approach with LVRS.[16–18] The IBV Valve trial (Spiration Valve System [SVS]) was a multicenter randomized sham-controlled, double-blind trial enrolling 277 subjects. Patients treated with partial bilateral upper lobe valve occlusion had a significant decrease in lobar volume compared with controls (224 mL vs 17 mL, respectively). The a priori primary outcome of disease-related quality of life, however, as measured by the SGRQ at 6 months, resulted in similar proportion of responders in the treatment and control groups. In addition, 14.1% of patients in the EBV treatment group experienced serious adverse events (SAEs) versus 3.7% in the control group.

A multicenter European Trial utilized partial occlusion of bilateral upper lobes and similarly demonstrated some improvement in lung volumes without improvement in SGRQ or exercise capacity.[16] These and other studies demonstrated that improvements in SGRQ were associated with greater volume decreases in the treated lobe (>350 mL) and subsequently that unilateral complete lobar occlusion was superior to bilateral partial lobar occlusion for quality of life improvement.[19,20] These and other data also highlighted the importance of achieving complete lobar atelectasis or lobar collapse with valve occlusion as a requisite for improved clinical response.[21]

LATER CLINICAL TRIALS

Subsequent trials concentrated on unilateral lobar occlusion rather than partial occlusion. The VENT [Endobronchial Valve for Emphysema Palliation Trial] trial was an early study comparing unilateral EBV therapy (Zephyr EBV, Pulmonx) versus standard medical care in 220 patients in patients with heterogeneous emphysema.[22] Although there were modest improvements in FEV$_1$ (mean improvement of 6.8% vs controls; P = .005) and 6MWD (mean improvement of 5.8% vs controls; P = .04), these were not determined to meet the MCID standard. Post hoc analysis of these data did, however, identify a subgroup of patients with intact interlobar fissures and patients with more prominent heterogeneity of disease that resulted in a much better response to EBV therapy.

Based on previous work, the BeLieVeR-HIFi study was a double-blind sham-controlled trial of 50 patients with heterogenous disease and intact interlobar fissures with the study cohort receiving complete target lobe occlusion with EBV.[9] HRCT was utilized to assess the degree of heterogeneity of disease and to identify target lobes with greater than 90% intact fissure by radiologist consensus. Although it was not utilized for patient stratification in the trial, the Chartis system was used in all patients to assess the degree of collateral ventilation and to compare to HRCT assessment of completeness of fissure.[23] This approach resulted in significant clinical improvements in FEV$_1$ and 6MWD at 3 months without differences in SGRQ. There were 4 patients in the EBV-treated cohort that were identified as having complete interlobar fissures by computed tomography (CT) assessment that were determined to have significant collateral ventilation by Chartis assessment. These 4 patients had no improvement in any parameters versus the control group, suggesting that better assessment of collateral ventilation might lead to better patient selection and improved efficacy.

The STELVIO trial evaluated patients with absence of collateral ventilation in the target lobe utilizing the Chartis system but was inclusive of patients with heterogeneous and homogeneous disease.[24] This resulted in exclusion of 13 patients because of Chartis identification of collateral ventilation. Among 68 patients randomized, FEV$_1$ at 6 months improved in the EBV group (161 mL vs 21 mL, mean difference 140 [55–225ml]; P = .002) versus controls with a 59% response rate in the EBV group versus 24% in the control group (P = .003). There also were improvements in FVC, increasing 6MWD by 74 m (P<.01), and a 14.7-point reduction in SGRQ with EBV. Post hoc analysis suggested relative improvements in FEV$_1$, RV, 6MWD, and SGRQ scores in patients with homogeneous disease versus controls, although these differences were not as pronounced as those in patients with heterogeneous disease.

The TRANSFORM trial randomized patients with only heterogeneous disease without collateral ventilation based on Chartis assessment.[25] In

Table 1
Clinical outcomes in randomized trials of endobronchial valve therapy for severe refractory emphysema

	N	Key Inclusion Criteria	Defined Follow-up Duration	Primary Endpoint	Treatment Arm	Forced Expiratory Volume in 1 Second (L)	Forced Expiratory Volume in 1 Second (>15%) Responders	St. George's Respiratory Questionnaire	St. George's Respiratory Questionnaire (0.4), Responders (%)	Six-Minute Walk Distance (m)	Six-Minute Walk Distance (>25 m), Responders (%)	Residual Volume (L)
VENT[22] Zephyr EBV vs SC	220	FEV$_1$ 15%–45% predicted; RV >150% predicted; TLC >100% predicted; 6MWD of ≥140 m; DLCO ≥20%	6 mo	% change in FEV$_1$%; Change in 6MWD	EBV	+0.034	23.5%	−2.8		+9.3	25.3	
					SC	−0.025	10.7%	+0.6		−10.7	17.8	NS
					Change	+0.060		−3.4		+19.1	NS	
IBV[16] SVS vs SC	72	FEV$_1$ ≤45% predicted; TLC ≥100% predicted; RV ≥150% predicted; 6MWD of ≥140 m; DLCO ≥20%	3 mo	Reduction in SGRQ total score ≥4; Change in CT measured lobar lung volume	EBV	−0.09				+7		+0.21
					SC	−0.01				+7		−0.21
					Change	−0.08 (NS)				NS		

Trial	N	Inclusion criteria	Follow-up	Outcome measure	Group							
IBV[18] SVS vs SC	277	FEV$_1$ ≤45% predicted; TLC ≥100% predicted; RV ≥150% predicted; 6MWD of ≥140 m	6 mo	Reduction in SGRQ total score ≥4; Change in CT measured lobar lung volume	EBV	−0.07		+2.15	32.2	−24.02		+0.31
					SC	0.00		−1.41	39.8	−3.4		−0.07
					Change			NS				
BeLieVeR-HIFi[9] Zephyr EBV vs SC	50	FEV$_1$ <50% predicted; TLC >100% predicted; RV >150% predicted; 6MWD < 450 m; MRC dyspnea Score ≥3	3 mo	% change in FEV$_1$%	EBV	+0.06	39%	−4.4	48	+25	52	−0.26
					SC	+0.03	4%	−3.57	46	+3	17	−0.08
					Change	+0.03		NS	NS	+22		+0.18 NS
STELVIO[24] Zephyr EBV vs SC	68	FEV$_1$ <60% predicted; TLC >100% predicted; RV >150% predicted; mMRC scale >1; Absence of collateral ventilation	6 mo	% difference from baseline for FEV$_1$, FVC and 6MWD from baseline	EBV	+0.161	59%	−21.8	79	+60	59	
					SC	+0.021	24%	−7.6	33	−14	6	
					Change	+0.14		−14.7		+74		

(continued on next page)

Table 1
(continued)

	N	Key Inclusion Criteria	Defined Follow-up Duration	Primary Endpoint	Treatment Arm	Forced Expiratory Volume in 1 Second (L)	Forced Expiratory Volume in 1 Second (>15% Responders)	St. George's Respiratory Questionnaire	St. George's Respiratory Questionnaire (0.4), Responders (%)	Six-Minute Walk Distance (m)	Six-Minute Walk Distance (>25 m), Responders (%)	Residual Volume (L)
IMPACT[27] Zephyr EBV vs SC	93	FEV_1 15%–45% predicted; RV ≥200% predicted; absence of collateral ventilation; Homogeneous emphysema	3 mo	% difference from baseline for FEV_1	EBV SC Change	+0.10 −0.02 +0.12	34.9% 4.0%	−8.63 +1.01 −9.64	56.8 25	+22.6 −17.3 +40	50 14	−0.42 +0.05 −0.48
TRAN-SFORM[25] Zephyr EBV vs SC	97	FEV_1 15%–45% predicted; RV ≥180% predicted; TLC >100% predicted; 6MWD 150–450 m; absence of collateral ventilation; Hetero-geneous emphysema	3 mo	FEV_1 ≥12% (% difference from baseline for FEV_1)	EBV SC Change	+0.14 −0.09 +0.23	56.3%[a] 3.2%	−7.2 −0.7 −6.5	61.7 34.4	+36.2 −42.5 +78.7	52.4 12.9	−0.66 +0.01 −0.67

Study	N	Inclusion criteria	Follow-up	Primary outcome	Group							
LIBERATE[26] Zephyr EBV vs SC	190	FEV_1 15%–45% predicted; RV ≥175% predicted; TLC >100% predicted; 6MWD 100–500 m; absence of collateral ventilation; heterogeneous emphysema	12 mo	FEV_1 ≥15% (% difference from baseline for FEV_1)	EBV	+0.104	47.7%	−7.55	56.2	+12.98	41.8	−0.49
					SC	−0.003	16.8%	−0.5	18	−26.33	19.6	+0.03
					Change	+0.106		−7.05		+39.31		−0.52
REACH[12] SVS vs SC	107	FEV_1 ≤45% predicted; TLC ≥100% predicted; RV ≥150% predicted; MRC dyspnea Score ≥2	3 mo	% change in FEV_1 % predicted;	EBV	+0.104	48%					−0.42
					SC	+0.003	13%					−0.08
					Change	+0.101						NS

(continued on next page)

Table 1
(continued)

	N	Key Inclusion Criteria	Defined Follow-up Duration	Primary Endpoint	Treatment Arm	Forced Expiratory Volume in 1 Second (L)	Forced Expiratory Volume in 1 Second (>15% Responders	St. George's Respiratory Question-naire	St. George's Respiratory Question-naire (0.4), Responders (%)	Six-Minute Walk Distance (m)	Six-Minute Walk Distance (>25 m), Resp-onders (%)	Residual Volume (L)
EMPROVE[11] SVS vs SC	172	FEV$_1$ < 45% predicted; RV ≥150% predicted; TLC ≥100% predicted; 6MWD ≥ 140 m; absence of collateral ventilation; Hetero-geneous emphysema	6 mo	FEV$_1$ ≥15% (% difference from baseline for FEV$_1$)	EBV	+0.099	36.8%	−8.1	54	−4.4	32.4	−0.402
					SC	−0.002	10%	+4.8	18	−11.3	22.9	−0.042
					Change	+0.101		−13		+6.9	NS	−0.361

Abbreviations: NS, not significant; SC, standard control group. VENT trial reported mean increase in RV of 0.69% for controls and 1.29% decrease in RV in EBV cohort (NS).
[a] FEV$_1$ greater than 12%.

this trial, lobes with the highest degree of destruction and lowest perfusion based on perfusion scintigraphy were considered the target lobes for EBV (Zephyr). These data demonstrated improvements in FEV_1, 6MWD, and SGRQ versus standard of care at 3 months and 6 months post-treatment.

Subsequently, the LIBERATE trial, the largest randomized trial with 12-month follow-up of both treatment arms, enrolled a similar population of patients with heterogeneous disease without collateral ventilation to evaluate the potential long-term impact of EBV treatment (Zephyr).[26] At 1 year, 48% of EBV-treated patients met the predefined MCID ($\geq$15% improvement in FEV_1) versus 17% for controls ($P<.001$). Further improvements were seen with 6MWD and SGRQ for EBV-treated patients out to a year. Secondary outcomes also demonstrated a decrease in the rate of respiratory failure events and a trend in reduction in hospitalization for COPD exacerbation with 1-year follow-up.

The REACH trial and the EMPROVE trial utilized the SVS to compare EBV therapy to standard medical therapy in patients with severe heterogeneous emphysema with intact or complete fissures based on HRCT with primary outcomes measured at 3 months and 6 months, respectively.[11,12] The REACH trial demonstrated improvements in mean FEV_1 with 48% experiencing a MCID greater than 15% at 3 months although there was no difference in 6MWD. The EMPROVE trial also demonstrated a mean improvement in FEV_1 at 6 months with a between group difference in MCID response rate (>15% improvement in FEV_1) of 25.7% at 6 months but similar to the REACH trial there was no improvement in 6MWD.[11] Similar trials using the Zephyr valve system, such as the LIBERATE trial, instituted pulmonary rehabilitation program after the valve procedure through the extent of the trial, which may have accounted for the improvements seen in 6MWD in that study, whereas in the EMPROVE study, whereas rehabilitation was required prior to study enrollment it was not instituted after the SVS valve placement. This highlights the importance of an aggressive pulmonary rehabilitation program in achieving clinical success, as was demonstrated with LVRS.

CLINICAL RESULTS IN HOMOGENEOUS DISEASE

Based on early data suggesting a potential benefit in patients with homogeneous disease, the IMPACT trial focused exclusively on patients with homogeneous disease. Although objective criteria for homogenous disease is limited, this was defined radiographically as less than 15% difference in emphysema destruction score between target and ipsilateral lobes.[22] Furthermore, less than 20% difference in perfusion between lungs was required based on perfusion scintigraphy. The target lobe for EBV (Zephyr) had the highest emphysema destruction score by HRCT, the lowest perfusion, and an absence of collateral ventilation. This resulted in selection of the left lower lobe as the target lobe in 42% of EBV-treated patients. With these criteria, EBV treatment resulted in a mean improvement in FEV_1 of 17% versus standard of care at 3 months.[27] There also was a 40-m mean improvement in the 6MWD, with 50% of patients in the EBV group having at least a 26-m improvement (MCID) versus 14% in controls ($P = .0002$). These data highlighted the importance of selecting low perfusion areas of lung for the greatest clinical benefit and helped potentially expand the pool of patients with COPD that might benefit from EBV treatment that essentially were excluded from surgical LVRS based on the NETT trial.

FUTURE TRIALS

As results have improved with EBV therapy, the question has arisen as to what the relative role of EBV is in relation to LVRS. The trial Comparative Effectiveness of Lung volume reduction surgery for Emphysema and Bronchoscopic lung volume reduction with valve placement (CELEB) is a randomized clinical trial designed to compare LVRS to BLVR with evaluation of clinical outcomes at 1 year. Key inclusion criteria for CELEB are FEV_1 less than 60% predicted, RV greater than 170% predicted, and heterogeneous disease with intact interlobar fissures. Surgical patients will undergo unilateral video assisted thoracoscopic surgery LVRS. The primary outcome at 1 year will be a composite COPD index, the iBODE score. The composite iBODE index includes incremental shuttle walk test, body mass index, FEV_1, and MRC dyspnea score.[28,29] A cost utility analysis also will be performed to compare the cost effectiveness of these therapies. This multicenter European trial began enrollment in October 2016 and should provide useful information regarding the relative efficacy of these therapies.[30]

COMPLICATIONS RELATED TO ENDOBRONCHIAL VALVE THERAPY

Although the motivation for pursuing EBV therapy was to potentially mitigate the morbidity and mortality reported with surgical LVRS, valve placement has not avoided some of the complications seen with volume reduction in these very-high-risk patients

Table 2
Complications of endobronchial valve therapy from randomized clinical trials for severe refractory emphysema

	N	Defined Follow-up Duration	Serious Adverse Events, N (%)	Pulmonary Infection, N (%)	Pneumo-thorax, N (%)	Valve Migration, N (%)	Valve Expec-toration, N (%)	Valve Dislo-cation, N (%)	Valve Removal, N (%)	Death, N (%)	Recurrent Nerve Paralysis, N (%)	Chronic Obstructive Pulmonary Disease Exacer-bation, N (%)	Hemo-ptysis, N (%)
VENT[22]	220/321	3 mo	9 (4.2)	4 (1.9)	9 (4.2)	10 (4.7)				2 (0.9)		20 (9.3)	12 (5.6)
IBV[16]	37/72	3 mo	7 (8)									11 (13)	1 (1)
IBV[18]	142/277	6 mo		1 (0.7)	3 (2.1)					6 (4.2)		7 (4.9)	
BeLieVeR-HIFi[9]	25/50	3 mo		2 (8)	2 (8)		5 (20)		2 (8)	2 (8)		16 (64)	
STELVIO[24]	34/68	6 mo	23	2 (6)	6 (18)	2 (6)		1 (3)		1 (3)			4 (12)
IMPACT[27]	43/93	3 mo	26 (44.2)		12 (25.6)	2 (4.6)				0	1 (2.3)	10 (16.3)	
TRANSFORM[25]	65/97	6 mo	35.2%	6 (9.2)	15 (23)				1 (1.5)			6 (9.2)	1 (1.5)
LIBERATE[26]	128/190	12 mo		8 (6.3)	44 (34.4)	3 (2)	2 (1.5)			5 (3.9)		38 (30)	
REACH[12]	66/107	6 mo	22 (33.3)		4 (6.1)					0		5 (7.6)	
EMPROVE[11]	113/172	6 mo	31%		29 (25.6)				11 (9.7)	6 (5.3)			

(Table 2). Treatment-related or 90-day mortality has remained low for EBV-treated patients, ranging from 1.2% to 3.1%,[9,11,12,16,22,24–27,31] in contrast to the NETT reported mortality of 5.2%. Some deaths are attributed to respiratory failure as might be anticipated based on the population, but deaths related to pneumothorax also have contributed to mortality in some studies.[24–26]

Pneumothorax has been a prominent and challenging complication associated with EBV therapy. Contemporary trials have reported a pneumothorax rate of 8% to 30% after valve insertion.[11,12,24–26,31] Early studies utilizing partial lobar occlusion techniques resulted in a lower incidence of pneumothorax with valve insertion but, as trials focused more on complete lobar occlusion in target lobes with limited collateral ventilation, the incidence of pneumothorax trended upward.[11,12,18,24–27,31] Many of these pneumothoraces occurred early after valve insertion with most occurring within the first 36 hours but several studies have reported delayed pneumothoraces ranging from 3 days to 14 days after valve insertion with some pneumothorax-related deaths. The development of pneumothoraces in these patients may be related to target lobe collapse, leading to compensatory rapid inflation of the diseased ipsilateral lobe. Management of post-treatment pneumothorax is similar to standard treatment of pneumothorax, with observation in some and chest tube placement if necessary, based on clinical assessment, although temporary or permanent removal of the valves also may be necessary for refractory pneumothoraces. Unfortunately, given the limited reserve in most of these patients, anticipation and early intervention are crucial to the perioperative management. Treatment guidelines have attempted to standardize the approach to these patients regarding pneumothorax risk and additional guidelines regarding length of hospitalization (ie, 3–5 days) also have been instituted because of the risk of delayed pneumothoraces in these patients.[11,26,32] Postdischarge pneumothorax remains a risk, however, making discharge planning and education a critical component of management of these patients.

The overall rate of SAEs has ranged from 25% to 48% among clinical trial data. Aside from pneumothorax and COPD exacerbation, other adverse events have included valve specific problems, such as torsion of the bronchus, postobstructive pneumonia, and intolerance of the valves related to cough and sputum production, requiring valve removal. Valve migration also may occur 2% to 6% of the time, requiring either valve revision or removal. Hemoptysis has been relatively uncommon after valve placement, although 1% to 2% but may require valve removal particularly if extensive granulation tissue develops around the valves.

OTHER ENDOBRONCHIAL THERAPIES

Endobronchial therapies other than EBV therapy have been developed to treat patients with severe COPD. Endobronchial coils are nonocclusive nitinol coils placed into subsegmental airways to induce parenchymal compression and enhance lung recoil. Coils are placed bronchoscopically with fluoroscopic guidance. Small clinical trials have demonstrated modest improvements in FEV_1, 6MWD, and SGRQ scores.[33–36] Consolidation and pneumonia in the target lobe have been more prominent than in the control groups, although it is possible that this consolidative effect may be related to the mechanism of coil compression and result in improved results in outcome variables. This mechanism is thought to be independent of collateral ventilation and potentially beneficial in patients with homogeneous disease. Further understanding of appropriate selection criteria, experience with coil insertion, and understanding of post-treatment radiographic findings may help improve the efficacy of coil therapy in the future. This therapy, however, currently is not approved for clinical use in the United States and also is not available outside the United States.

Bronchoscopy thermal vapor ablation (BTVA) utilizes thermal energy to induce an inflammatory process in the target lobe, resulting in atelectasis and fibrosis of the diseased lung tissue to invoke lung volume reduction. Similar to coil therapy, early trials have demonstrated modest improvements in primary clinical outcomes; however, COPD exacerbations and pneumonitis have plagued these patients[37]; like the coils, BTVA currently is not approved for clinical use in the United States. Lung sealants or sclerosants also have been developed to be bronchoscopically injected into hyperinflated segments to induce atelectasis in the diseased lobe (AeriSeal Emphysematous Lung Sealant, Pulmonx). This therapy was associated with significant SAEs requiring hospitalization in 44% of the treated cohort and is not approved for clinical use in the United States at this time.[38]

SUMMARY

EBV therapy has evolved rapidly over the past decade, with clinical responses that potentially rival or approach the clinical response seen with surgical LVRS. It is clear that careful patient selection is critical with meticulous work-up to identify the target lobe with the most significant disease and limited or no collateral ventilation. Achievement of lobar collapse is requisite for the best clinical response but also may result in a higher risk of pneumothorax. Based on the current data, EBV potentially may be considered in patients that are candidates for surgical LVRS, although direct comparative studies have not been completed. On the other hand, EBV therapy may benefit other subsets of patients with COPD who would not have been considered for LVRS because of the distribution of their disease. The benefit seen in patients with homogeneous disease may expand treatment options in these difficult patients with limited options. Although LVRS has been the standard of care in appropriately selected patients, the evolution of EBV therapy provides a valuable alternative tool in the treatment of severe emphysema, and, as this therapy continues to improve with patient selection and mitigation of complications, EBV certainly will play a dominant role in the future management of these patients.

CLINICS CARE POINTS

- EBV therapy results in significant improvement in FEV_1, 6MWD, and quality of life among patients with end-stage COPD

- Reported rates of pneumothorax after EBV insertion range from 8% to 30% and may occur early or in a delayed fashion.

- EBV therapy may be beneficial in select patients with homogeneous emphysema with improvements in FEV_1, 6MWDp, and quality of life.

DISCLOSURE

No financial disclosures.

REFERENCES

1. Habraken JM, van der Wal WM, Ter Riet G, et al. Health-related quality of life and functional status in end-stage COPD: a longitudinal study. Eur Respir J 2011;37(2):280–8.
2. Cooper JD, Trulock EP, Triantafillou AN, et al. Bilateral pneumectomy (volume reduction) for chronic obstructive pulmonary disease. J Thorac Cardiovasc Surg 1995;109(1):106–16 [discussion: 116–9].
3. Fishman A, Martinez F, Naunheim K, et al. A randomized trial comparing lung-volume-reduction surgery with medical therapy for severe emphysema. N Engl J Med 2003;348(21):2059–73.
4. Naunheim KS, Wood DE, Mohsenifar Z, et al. Long-term follow-up of patients receiving lung-volume-reduction surgery versus medical therapy for severe emphysema by the National Emphysema Treatment Trial Research Group. Ann Thorac Surg 2006;82(2):431–43.
5. McNulty W, Jordan S, Hopkinson NS. Attitudes and access to lung volume reduction surgery for COPD: a survey by the British Thoracic Society. BMJ Open Respir Res 2014;1(1):e000023.
6. Tuohy MM, Remund KF, Hilfiker R, et al. Endobronchial valve deployment in severe alpha-1 antitrypsin deficiency emphysema: a case series. Clin Respir J 2013;7(1):45–52.
7. Hillerdal G, Mindus S. One- to four-year follow-up of endobronchial lung volume reduction in alpha-1-antitrypsin deficiency patients: a case series. Respiration 2014;88(4):320–8.
8. Eberhardt R, Herth FJ, Radhakrishnan S, et al. Comparing clinical outcomes in upper versus lower lobe endobronchial valve treatment in severe emphysema. Respiration 2015;90(4):314–20.
9. Davey C, Zoumot Z, Jordan S, et al. Bronchoscopic lung volume reduction with endobronchial valves for patients with heterogeneous emphysema and intact interlobar fissures (the BeLieVeR-HIFi study): a randomised controlled trial. Lancet 2015;386(9998):1066–73.
10. Herth FJ, Eberhardt R, Gompelmann D, et al. Radiological and clinical outcomes of using Chartis to plan endobronchial valve treatment. Eur Respir J 2013;41(2):302–8.
11. Criner GJ, Delage A, Voelker K, et al. Improving lung function in severe heterogenous emphysema with the spiration valve system (EMPROVE). a multicenter, open-label randomized controlled clinical trial. Am J Respir Crit Care Med 2019;200(11):1354–62.
12. Li S, Wang G, Wang C, et al. The REACH trial: a randomized controlled trial assessing the safety and effectiveness of the spiration(R) valve system in the treatment of severe emphysema. Respiration 2019;97(5):416–27.
13. Donohue JF. Minimal clinically important differences in COPD lung function. COPD 2005;2(1):111–24.
14. Jones PW. St. George's respiratory questionnaire: MCID. COPD 2005;2(1):75–9.
15. Puhan MA, Chandra D, Mosenifar Z, et al. The minimal important difference of exercise tests in severe COPD. Eur Respir J 2011;37(4):784–90.
16. Ninane V, Geltner C, Bezzi M, et al. Multicentre European study for the treatment of advanced emphysema with bronchial valves. Eur Respir J 2012;39(6):1319–25.
17. Wood DE, McKenna RJ Jr, Yusen RD, et al. A multicenter trial of an intrabronchial valve for treatment of severe emphysema. J Thorac Cardiovasc Surg 2007;133(1):65–73.

18. Wood DE, Nader DA, Springmeyer SC, et al. The IBV Valve trial: a multicenter, randomized, double-blind trial of endobronchial therapy for severe emphysema. J Bronchology Interv Pulmonol 2014; 21(4):288–97.

19. Eberhardt R, Gompelmann D, Schuhmann M, et al. Complete unilateral vs partial bilateral endoscopic lung volume reduction in patients with bilateral lung emphysema. Chest 2012;142(4):900–8.

20. Herth FJ, Noppen M, Valipour A, et al. Efficacy predictors of lung volume reduction with Zephyr valves in a European cohort. Eur Respir J 2012;39(6): 1334–42.

21. Hopkinson NS, Kemp SV, Toma TP, et al. Atelectasis and survival after bronchoscopic lung volume reduction for COPD. Eur Respir J 2011;37(6): 1346–51.

22. Sciurba FC, Ernst A, Herth FJ, et al. A randomized study of endobronchial valves for advanced emphysema. N Engl J Med 2010;363(13):1233–44.

23. Shah PL, Herth FJ. Dynamic expiratory airway collapse and evaluation of collateral ventilation with Chartis. Thorax 2014;69(3):290–1.

24. Klooster K, ten Hacken NH, Hartman JE, et al. Endobronchial valves for emphysema without interlobar collateral ventilation. N Engl J Med 2015;373(24): 2325–35.

25. Kemp SV, Slebos DJ, Kirk A, et al. A multicenter randomized controlled trial of zephyr endobronchial valve treatment in heterogeneous emphysema (TRANSFORM). Am J Respir Crit Care Med 2017; 196(12):1535–43.

26. Criner GJ, Sue R, Wright S, et al. A multicenter randomized controlled trial of zephyr endobronchial valve treatment in heterogeneous emphysema (LIBERATE). Am J Respir Crit Care Med 2018; 198(9):1151–64.

27. Valipour A, Slebos DJ, Herth F, et al. Endobronchial valve therapy in patients with homogeneous emphysema. results from the IMPACT study. Am J Respir Crit Care Med 2016;194(9):1073–82.

28. Hakamy A, McKeever TM, Steiner MC, et al. The use of the practice walk test in pulmonary rehabilitation program: National COPD Audit Pulmonary Rehabilitation Workstream. Int J Chron Obstruct Pulmon Dis 2017;12:2681–6.

29. Williams JE, Green RH, Warrington V, et al. Development of the i-BODE: validation of the incremental shuttle walking test within the BODE index. Respir Med 2012;106(3):390–6.

30. Buttery S, Kemp SV, Shah PL, et al. CELEB trial: Comparative Effectiveness of Lung volume reduction surgery for Emphysema and Bronchoscopic lung volume reduction with valve placement: a protocol for a randomised controlled trial. BMJ Open 2018;8(10):e021368.

31. Fiorelli A, D'Andrilli A, Bezzi M, et al. Complications related to endoscopic lung volume reduction for emphysema with endobronchial valves: results of a multicenter study. J Thorac Dis 2018;10(Suppl 27): S3315–25.

32. Valipour A, Slebos DJ, de Oliveira HG, et al. Expert statement: pneumothorax associated with endoscopic valve therapy for emphysema–potential mechanisms, treatment algorithm, and case examples. Respiration 2014;87(6):513–21.

33. Deslee G, Mal H, Dutau H, et al. Lung volume reduction coil treatment vs usual care in patients with severe emphysema: the REVOLENS randomized clinical trial. JAMA 2016;315(2):175–84.

34. Sciurba FC, Chandra D, Bon J. Bronchoscopic lung volume reduction in COPD: lessons in implementing clinically based precision medicine. JAMA 2016; 315(2):139–41.

35. Sciurba FC, Criner GJ, Strange C, et al. Effect of endobronchial coils vs usual care on exercise tolerance in patients with severe emphysema: the RENEW randomized clinical trial. JAMA 2016; 315(20):2178–89.

36. Shah PL, Zoumot Z, Singh S, et al. Endobronchial coils for the treatment of severe emphysema with hyperinflation (RESET): a randomised controlled trial. Lancet Respir Med 2013;1(3):233–40.

37. Herth FJ, Valipour A, Shah PL, et al. Segmental volume reduction using thermal vapour ablation in patients with severe emphysema: 6-month results of the multicentre, parallel-group, open-label, randomised controlled STEP-UP trial. Lancet Respir Med 2016;4(3):185–93.

38. Come CE, Kramer MR, Dransfield MT, et al. A randomised trial of lung sealant versus medical therapy for advanced emphysema. Eur Respir J 2015;46(3):651–62.

Lung Volume Reduction Surgery in Patients with Homogeneous Emphysema

Walter Weder, MD[a],*, Laurens J. Ceulemans, MD, PhD[b], Isabelle Opitz, MD[c],
Didier Schneiter, MD[c], Claudio Caviezel, MD[c]

KEYWORDS

- LVRS • Homogeneous emphysema • Surgery for emphysema

KEY POINTS

- Lung volume reduction surgery (LVRS) offers clinical and functional benefit in hyperinflated patients with homogeneous-type emphysema. It is important to exclude patients with low diffusing capacity of the lungs for carbon monoxide or pulmonary hypertension.
- LVRS in patients with homogeneous emphysema requires more experience with LVRS than in patients with heterogenous disease with obvious target zones for resection.
- The functional benefit of LVRS in homogeneous emphysema is clinically relevant but smaller than in heterogenous emphysema.

INTRODUCTION

Lung volume reduction surgery (LVRS) improves pulmonary function, exercise capacity, quality of life, and even survival in highly selected patients with advanced emphysema.[1–4] Almost all of these studies, including the largest randomized trial comparing LVRS with medical therapy, the National Emphysema Treatment Trial, obtain their successful results from operated patients with heterogeneous emphysema morphology. The argument, that in patients with heterogeneous emphysema only nonperfused, functionless tissue is resected, is convincing. Furthermore, this target area for resection is clearly identifiable on computed tomographic (CT) scan and perfusion scintigraphy. Especially in the case of upper lobe predominant emphysema, resection and remodeling of the lung are easy and straightforward.

The idea, to resect tissue with remaining gas-exchange function in patients with poor lung function owing to homogeneously situated emphysema, is difficult to justify. Nevertheless,

with respect to certain selection criteria, promising results about LVRS in patients with homogeneous emphysema are reported. The first larger study on this subgroup demonstrated significant benefit after surgery, although results are slightly inferior compared with LVRS in heterogeneous emphysema.[5] Despite this positive report, most other centers continued to exclude patients with homogeneous emphysema from their program. This negative attitude was further supported by a publication from the National Emphysema Treatment Trial (NETT), which described a very high mortality after LVRS in patients with a homogeneous morphology. However, these patients with homogeneous diffuse emphysema had a heavily destroyed (vanished) lung with very low forced expiratory values in 1 second (FEV1 <20% predicted) and a diffusion capacity less than 20% predicted. This report was misinterpreted by many physicians, which concluded that all patients experience a high mortality after LVRS.[6,7] However, it was shown that patients from the NETT with homogeneous emphysema in combination with

[a] Thoracic Surgery, Thoraxchirurgie Bethanien, Toblerstrasse 61, 8044 Zürich, Switzerland; [b] Department of Thoracic Surgery, University Hospitals Leuven, Herestraat 49, 3000 Leuven, Belgium; [c] Department of Thoracic Surgery, University Hospital Zürich, Rämistrasse 100, 8091 Zürich, Switzerland
* Corresponding author.
E-mail address: w.weder@thorax-zuerich.ch

Thorac Surg Clin 31 (2021) 203–209
https://doi.org/10.1016/j.thorsurg.2021.02.007
1547-4127/21/© 2021 Elsevier Inc. All rights reserved.

FEV1 greater than 20% predicted and diffusion capacity greater than 20% predicted had a significant improvement of certain pulmonary function parameters as well.[8]

Nevertheless, lung volume reduction (LVR) in homogenous emphysema type has been avoided by most groups for a long time. With the emergence of bronchoscopic LVR techniques, new attempts to improve dyspnea also in patients with homogeneous morphology were undertaken, and the results were reported.

Therefore, this review discusses the rationale of LVR, the definition of homogeneous emphysema, the selection process, management, and outcome after LVRS as well as the bronchoscopic treatment. Outcomes are summarized, leading to a recommendation, and an attempt to stimulate other groups to offer LVRS in well-selected patients. Clinical scenarios will be used to illustrate the daily practice in the decision process and management of patients.

RATIONALE BEHIND LUNG VOLUME REDUCTION

Emphysema is a loss of pulmonary elasticity by destruction of alveolar walls and capillaries and by enlarged airways distal to the terminal bronchioles. The consequence of the latter is lung hyperinflation, which interferes with respiratory mechanics, among other physiologic changes. Primarily, the diaphragm is pressed down, and the suspension of the muscle fibers becomes almost perpendicular, which inhibits full function. Volume reduction intends to re-create the normal lung volume (total lung capacity [TLC]) and reshapes the lung to its original form.[9] LVRS allows an individual remodeling of the lungs, by selecting the target areas for resection based on emphysema morphology on CT and perfusion scans. With the gained intrathoracic space, the diaphragm might return to its original position, and even more importantly, to its domelike shape. The residual volume (RV) is reduced, and the lung's elastic recoil is improved. The diaphragm regains more strength and work capacity, which improves breath work and decreases dyspnea.[10] In addition, airflow improves by reopening the collapsed small airways because of reinstalled pull-out forces. The same effect leads to opening of capillaries, which reduces the ventilation/perfusion mismatch and improves diffusion capacity, and hence, might decrease pulmonary hypertension.[11]

Reducing hyperinflation in emphysema treatment seems to be the most important step. In 1 randomized controlled trial, although shown with the meanwhile abandoned endobronchial coils compared with medical treatment, improvements in lung function, quality of life, and 6-minute walking distance were significantly better, when performed in patients with RV greater than 225% than in patients with RV between 175% and 225%.[12] Most concerns about LVR(S) in homogeneous emphysema might arise from the fear of resecting (or bypassing, respectively) functional tissue, which contributes to gas exchange. Obvious target areas of complete destruction for resection are lacking. Therefore, in an adequate volume resection, it is important to balance the positive effect of improved respiratory mechanics with the disadvantage of resecting functional tissue of gas exchange. LVR with endobronchial valves in homogeneous emphysema showed some positive effect, although the downside of this minimally invasive LVR technique is that consequently a whole lobe is eliminated.[13] In contrast, surgery offers a more tailored approach, as the "homogeneous" emphysema type allows the identification often of some "intermediate" parts of destruction, when carefully assessed with appropriate imaging methods like CT in combination with densitometry.[14] In addition, in purely homogeneous emphysema, the surgeon might approach both apical parts of the upper lobes, which are usually physiologically less perfused and therefore less effective for gas exchange.

DEFINITION OF HOMOGENEOUS EMPHYSEMA

One of the major challenges of homogeneous emphysema is its definition. There are different proposals to define homogeneity in emphysema morphology. All of them were basically developed from either a surgical or an interventional point of view and are difficult to compare.

One of the first definitions of emphysema morphology, including homogeneous emphysema, was CT based and has been introduced more than 20 years ago with the intention to get a simple and practical guide for patient selection for LVRS and for comparison of results.[14] The markedly heterogeneous emphysema, including upper-lobe or lower-lobe predominance with and without the apical segments of the lower lobes, was differentiated from intermediately heterogeneous and homogeneous emphysema. Intermediately heterogeneous emphysema includes an anatomically indistinct subgroup that might look like homogeneous on the first view, but when studied carefully, several target areas of smaller size for LVRS can be identified (**Fig. 1**). Summarized with an adagium: "The longer you look to homogeneous emphysema, the more heterogeneous it becomes." The purely homogeneous emphysema

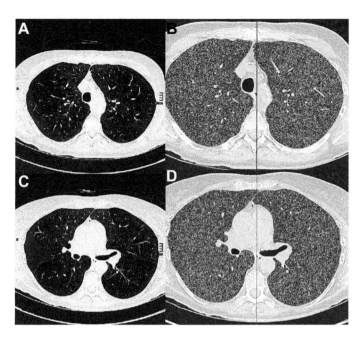

Fig. 1. Bilateral intermediate heterogeneous emphysema. Several potential target zones become obvious by densitometry. Lateral upper lobe on the right side: (*A*) axial CT scan, (*B*) densitometry, segment 6 on the right side: (*C*) axial CT scan, (*D*) densitometry.

itself, as long as CT, perfusion scintigraphy, and (if available) densitometric measurements are meticulously analyzed, offers no target area of distinct destruction (**Fig. 2**). The identification and classification of emphysema morphology are based on eye-balling slice by slice the CT scan. However, certain software applications allow density measurements that can be transferred in colored CT pictures, which might be useful for identifying different morphologies, such as pure homogeneity.[15] These so-called color-coded CT renderings offer additional aspects for the surgeon in planning target zones for LVRS.[16]

The investigators of the IMPACT trial defined homogeneous emphysema as a less than 15% difference in emphysema destruction score between target and ipsilateral lobes in a study using bronchoscopic LVR with endobronchial valves.[13] They used CT quantitative analysis software to measure volumes and destruction. These measurements regarding the density differences were performed using −910 HU as margin. In addition, less than 20% perfusion difference between both lung sides was required. For the IMPACT study, both criteria had to be met.

In the literature, some investigators use the term "diffuse" or homogeneous for any type of advanced emphysema, but are actually reporting LVRS in patients with heterogeneous emphysema; this insight might be clearer if one carefully reads the methods section of some reports.[10,17] The term diffuse emphysema should be avoided in the future.

PATIENT SELECTION

Symptomatic patients with advanced emphysema and the typical clinical signs of hyperinflation are potential candidates for LVRS. Their barrel-like chest, tendency to pause their walks and rest their arms, and their inability to eat large meals must be further assessed with pulmonary function test and body plethysmography. Facing a patient with both clinical and body plethysmographic hyperinflation at least (RV >180%, TLC >100%, RV/TLC >58) seems in the authors' experience to be the key to success. Patients with so-called dynamic hyperinflation (not obviously seen on static measurements) might be considered for LVR(S) as well, despite the current lack of scientific support. This finding needs further investigation.[18] Comorbidities and pulmonary as well as nonpulmonary risk factors must be taken into account and balanced with the risk and potential benefit.

Emphysema morphology assessed by CT and perfusion scan is of great importance for selecting patients. This selection of patients is especially important when patients have a more homogeneous pattern. In these cases, lung tissue, which still contributes to gas exchange, will be resected, or in the case of valve placement, an entire lobe is excluded. Therefore, a low CO-perfusion capacity or pulmonary hypertension is an absolute contraindication in homogeneous emphysema.

Although there is emerging evidence about successful LVRS in patients with mild to moderate pulmonary hypertension,[11] so far this combination

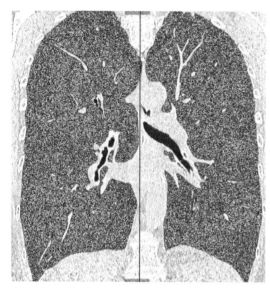

Fig. 2. Purely homogeneous emphysema without obvious target zones for LVRS (coronal densitometry).

probably needs to be restricted to patients with markedly heterogeneous emphysema. In these cases, only the nonperfused lung parts are resected, so that the elastic recoil of the parts contributing to diffusion is improved. The same shall be true for patients with very low diffusion capacity (<20%) or global respiratory insufficiency.[19] A transthoracic screening echocardiography can be advised, followed by further investigation by right-sided heart catheter when systolic pulmonary artery pressure (sPAP) is greater than 35 mm Hg.

A very low diffusion capacity was a significant risk factor for postsurgical 30-day mortality during the NETT trial, but importantly, in combination with homogeneous emphysema or FEV1 less than 20%.[6] Emphysema morphology was visually assessed by radiologists, dividing the lung into 3 zones. It remains unclear how many of the included 46 homogeneous emphysema types could have been counted as intermediately heterogeneous. They might still have profited by offering a tailored surgical approach, not just by the usual during the NETT performed upper-lobe-targeted "over-the-top," hockey-stick resection.

Other pulmonary risk factors, such as large airway disease or scarring of the parenchyma detected on CT, are absolute contraindications in these patients.

However, LVRS can be offered to every emphysema type, by careful patient selection. The decision is made based on a synopsis of patient factors, physiologic parameters, and emphysema morphology. **Table 1** lists inclusion criteria for patients with purely homogeneous emphysema.

RESULTS OF SURGICAL LUNG VOLUME REDUCTION IN HOMOGENEOUS EMPHYSEMA

Weder and colleagues[5] published the largest series on homogeneous emphysema in a single-center series of 250 consecutively operated patients, including 138 homogeneous emphysema types. From these, 82 had an intermediate morphology (see above). Results for patients with either intermediate or purely homogeneous emphysema were similar, and therefore, both were summarized as homogeneous. For the latter, 3 months after LVRS, FEV1% predicted improvement by 35% from 28 to 38, 6-minute walking distance improved from 245 to 324 m, and dyspnea score decreased from 3.5 to 1.8 (P<.05 for all outcomes). Median time until most values had returned to baseline was 36 months in both the heterogeneous and the homogeneous group. Thirty-day mortality was 2.4% for both groups, as well as 1-year survival was similar. Median survival after 5 years without lung transplantation was 64% in the homogeneous and 73% in the heterogeneous group. Regarding lung function in the heterogeneous group, FEV1% predicted increased from 29 to 44 (52% improvement), 6-minute walking distance from 243 to 382 m, and dyspnea score from 3.5 to 1.3.

Marchetti and colleagues[8] looked at the NETT data, comparing 85 patients with homogeneous emphysema and endobronchial coil treatment from 3 randomized trials from 2012, 2013, and 2014 with 51 patients from the NETT trial from 2003. In addition, 43 patients with medical treatment from the NETT were compared as well. Patients were matched regarding spirometry, age, and gender. LVRS patients were significantly older (64 vs 61 years, P<.01), had a worse baseline diffusion capacity (26.1 vs 33.4%, P<.01), but had a better baseline 6-minute walking distance (371 vs 311 m, P<.01).

The same definition for homogeneous emphysema from the NETT, as mentioned above, was applied.

At 6 months, no significant differences for FEV1 were detected between groups. There was a significant decrease in RV (P = .002) and TLC (P<.001) in both the coils and the LVRS group compared with medical therapy. The magnitude of the decline in both values was greater in the LVRS group. At 12 months, there remained a significant decline in RV (P = .006) and TLC (P<.001) compared with baseline in both groups compared with medical therapy.

Morbidity and mortality after LVRS seem still to be an issue comparing the different LVR techniques. The 90-day mortality from the NETT trial continues to be cited,[20] although carefully selected

Table 1
Inclusion and exclusion criteria for lung volume reduction surgery in patients with purely homogeneous emphysema

Criteria	Inclusion	Exclusion
Patient	Nicotine abstention >4 mo	Daily steroid intake >20 mg
Lung function	FEV <45% RV >180% TLC >100%	FEV1 <20% and/or DLCO <20%
6-min walking distance		>600 m
Gas exchange		$Paco_2$ >6.7 Pa and Pao_2 <6.0 Pa ($Paco_2$ >50 mm Hg and Pao_2 <45 mm Hg)
Pulmonary pressure		mPAP >35 mm Hg (right heart catheter)

Abbreviation: DLCO, diffusing capacity of the lungs for carbon monoxide; mPAP, median pulmonary artery pressure.

patient cohorts have shown much lower rates. The mortality of 5.2% in 511 patients[1] went down to 4.8% in 250 patients from Ciccone and colleagues,[2] to 2.4% in 250 patients from Weder and colleagues,[4] and even to 0 in 91 patients from Ginsburg and colleagues.[3] The series of Weder even included 138 patients with homogeneous emphysema, which had the same surgical mortality.

RESULTS OF BRONCHOSCOPIC LUNG VOLUME REDUCTION IN HOMOGENEOUS EMPHYSEMA

Despite initially somehow promising results, endobronchial coils for emphysema treatment have now been abandoned.[21–23] The focus has shifted toward one-way endobronchial valves, which originally have been used in heterogeneous emphysema only. The IMPACT trial randomized 43 patients with homogeneous emphysema and without collateral ventilation treated with valves versus 50 patients with medical standard care alone.[13] For the LVR group, absolute median improvement of FEV1 at 3 months compared with baseline was 100 mL. The median 6-minute walking distance improved by 23 m. From all endobronchially treated patients, 26% developed a pneumothorax with requirement for urgent chest tube treatment, and 11.5% needed some sort of revision bronchoscopy. Although difficult to compare, most studies report rates of prolonged air leak (defined as longer than 7 days) after LVRS of about 25% to 45%.[19]

SURGICAL CONCEPTS
Patient with Purely Homogeneous Emphysema

Patients with no obvious target zones on CT scan, perfusion scintigraphy, and densitometry but

relevant hyperinflation might be operated bilaterally (see **Fig. 2**). The authors recommend a supine position with both arms raised. The operation is always initiated as video-assisted thoracoscopic surgery (VATS). With the patient in the supine position, both sides can be approached from the anterolateral position without changing the patient's position. This approach is feasible for bilateral upper-lobe "over-the-top" resections. For lower-lobe resection, the lateral decubitus position is recommended as well as lowering the placement of the ports by 2 to 3 intercostal regions.

The operation would be prematurely terminated in case the first side would need extensive adhesiolysis with consecutive unavoidable air leak.

Patient with Side Predominance and/or Intermediate (Heterogeneous) Emphysema

Lungs with intermediate emphysema morphology often require more than 1 resection area and often involve at least 2 lobes or only the middle and lower lobes (see **Fig. 1**). The patient is placed in the lateral decubitus position, and the VATS approach is performed as for other (ie, anatomic) resections. When the operation is planned to be bilateral and the first side is successfully done, the patient's position is changed.

In cases of unilateral disease predominance, the LVRS is performed unilaterally (**Fig. 3**).

Patient after Unilateral Bronchoscopic Lung Volume Reduction with Valves

Patients are referred more often for LVRS after a first primary or secondary unsuccessful LVR procedure, including endobronchial valve placement. There is so far no evidence whether these valves should be removed or not before LVRS. The authors' experience[24] points toward an

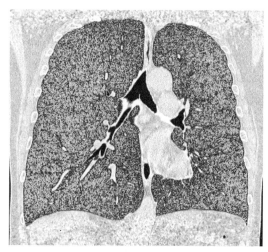

Fig. 3. Homogeneous emphysema with predominance on the right side (coronal densitometry); a unilateral procedure is suggested.

individualized approach: Valves with persistent atelectasis should not be removed and LVRS should be performed on the contralateral side. Valves without or with loss of atelectasis should be removed, as the initial target zone might be ideal for surgical resection as well (see **Fig. 3**).

SUMMARY AND RECOMMENDATIONS

Allocating patients to LVRS and selecting the adequate amount of tissue to be resected must be considered carefully in the presence of homogeneous disease. Because the main clinical effect derives from improved respiratory mechanics and because the resected tissue is still contributing to gas exchange, the presence of relevant hyperinflation is of paramount importance on 1 side. The other key element is absence of a "vanished" lung (identified by low gas exchange and/or pulmonary hypertension). These factors are the 2 key factors when considering homogeneous emphysema for LVRS.

Indication for LVRS depends on many factors, and therefore, it is impossible to give clear, straightforward recommendations that can be applied to all patients. Indication is a synopsis of clinical factors, physiologic parameters, and most importantly, the emphysema morphology assessed on CT and perfusion scan. Markedly heterogeneous emphysema includes an obvious target zone for resection. In these circumstances, by resection of only functionless, hyperinflated tissue, even borderline patients with severely impaired diffusion capacity and/or with mild to moderate pulmonary hypertension often can be accepted. In return, the exclusion criteria list is

more complex and must consider the balance between reducing hyperinflation and resecting tissue, which still contributes to gas exchange.

Once the patient is suitable for LVRS, the surgeon must have a clear concept of the operation. In diffuse homogeneity, a bilateral upper-lobe "over-the-top" approach should be performed, in the authors' opinion. In cases with intermediate morphology, different imaging techniques are advisable to detect potential target zones with less function. Patients with marked side differences might profit from a unilateral approach.

CLINICS CARE POINTS

- Select patients with homogenous emphysema for lung volume reduction surgery only, when the lungs are severely hyperinflated and the diaphragm is flat.

- Diffusing capacity of the lungs for carbon monoxide must be more than 20% to 30% when lung volume reduction surgery is planned in homogenous disease.

- Remodeling of the lungs by downsizing to its predicted volume is best done at the upper lobes by resecting a hockey-stick piece.

- The lungs must be semi-inflated in order to estimate the volume you want to resect during video-assisted thoracoscopic surgery.

DISCLOSURE

W. Weder: Astra Zeneca: Advisory Board & Speaker, Covidien (Medtronic): Teaching Grant & Speaker.

REFERENCES

1. Fishman A, Martinez F, Naunheim K, et al. A randomized trial comparing lung-volume-reduction surgery with medical therapy for severe emphysema. N Engl J Med 2003;348(21):2059–73.
2. Ciccone AM, Meyers BF, Guthrie TJ, et al. Long-term outcome of bilateral lung volume reduction in 250 consecutive patients with emphysema. J Thorac Cardiovasc Surg 2003;125(3):513–25.
3. Ginsburg ME, Thomashow BM, Bulman WA, et al. The safety, efficacy, and durability of lung-volume reduction surgery: a 10-year experience. J Thorac Cardiovasc Surg 2016;151(3):717–724 e1.

4. Tutic M, Lardinois D, Imfeld S, et al. Lung-volume reduction surgery as an alternative or bridging procedure to lung transplantation. Ann Thorac Surg 2006;82(1):208–13 [discussion: 13].

5. Weder W, Tutic M, Lardinois D, et al. Persistent benefit from lung volume reduction surgery in patients with homogeneous emphysema. Ann Thorac Surg 2009;87(1):229–36 [discussion: 36–7].

6. National Emphysema Treatment Trial Research Group, Fishman A, Fessler H, Martinez F, et al. Patients at high risk of death after lung-volume-reduction surgery. N Engl J Med 2001;345(15): 1075–83.

7. Criner GJ, Cordova F, Sternberg AL, et al. The National Emphysema Treatment Trial (NETT) Part II: lessons learned about lung volume reduction surgery. Am J Respir Crit Care Med 2011;184(8):881–93.

8. Marchetti N, Kaufman T, Chandra D, et al. Endobronchial coils versus lung volume reduction surgery or medical therapy for treatment of advanced homogenous emphysema. Chronic Obstr Pulm Dis 2018;5(2):87–96.

9. Cassart M, Hamacher J, Verbandt Y, et al. Effects of lung volume reduction surgery for emphysema on diaphragm dimensions and configuration. Am J Respir Crit Care Med 2001;163(5):1171–5.

10. Sciurba FC, Rogers RM, Keenan RJ, et al. Improvement in pulmonary function and elastic recoil after lung-reduction surgery for diffuse emphysema. N Engl J Med 1996;334(17):1095–9.

11. Caviezel C, Aruldas C, Franzen D, et al. Lung volume reduction surgery in selected patients with emphysema and pulmonary hypertension. Eur J Cardiothorac Surg 2018;54(3):565–71.

12. Sciurba FC, Criner GJ, Strange C, et al. Effect of endobronchial coils vs usual care on exercise tolerance in patients with severe emphysema: the RENEW randomized clinical trial. JAMA 2016; 315(20):2178–89.

13. Valipour A, Slebos DJ, Herth F, et al. Endobronchial valve therapy in patients with homogeneous emphysema. Results from the IMPACT study. Am J Respir Crit Care Med 2016;194(9):1073–82.

14. Weder W, Thurnheer R, Stammberger U, et al. Radiologic emphysema morphology is associated with outcome after surgical lung volume reduction. Ann Thorac Surg 1997;64(2):313–9 [discussion: 9–20].

15. Caviezel CFT, Schneiter D, Muehlmatter U, et al. Identification of target zones for lung volume reduction surgery using three-dimensional computed tomography rendering. Eur Respir J Open Res 2020; 6(3). 00305-2020 accepted June 04, 2020.

16. Muehlematter UJ, Caviezel C, Martini K, et al. Applicability of color-coded computed tomography images in lung volume reduction surgery planning. J Thorac Dis 2019;11(3):766–76.

17. Wisser W, Tschernko E, Wanke T, et al. Functional improvements in ventilatory mechanics after lung volume reduction surgery for homogeneous emphysema. Eur J Cardiothorac Surg 1997;12(4): 525–30.

18. Straub G, Caviezel C, Frauenfelder T, et al. Successful lung volume reduction surgery in combined pulmonary emphysema and fibrosis without body-plethysmographic hyperinflation-a case report. J Thorac Dis 2018;10(Suppl 23):S2830–4.

19. Caviezel C, Schaffter N, Schneiter D, et al. Outcome after lung volume reduction surgery in patients with severely impaired diffusion capacity. Ann Thorac Surg 2018;105(2):379–85.

20. Gompelmann D. Hope for patients with homogeneous emphysema? Chronic Obstr Pulm Dis 2018; 5(2):84–6.

21. Shah PL, Zoumot Z, Singh S, et al. Endobronchial coils for the treatment of severe emphysema with hyperinflation (RESET): a randomised controlled trial. Lancet Respir Med 2013;1(3):233–40.

22. Deslee G, Klooster K, Hetzel M, et al. Lung volume reduction coil treatment for patients with severe emphysema: a European multicentre trial. Thorax 2014;69(11):980–6.

23. Slebos DJ, Klooster K, Ernst A, et al. Bronchoscopic lung volume reduction coil treatment of patients with severe heterogeneous emphysema. Chest 2012; 142(3):574–82.

24. Caviezel C, Guglielmetti LC, Ladan M, et al. Lung volume reduction surgery as salvage procedure after previous use of endobronchial valves. Interact Cardiovasc Thorac Surg 2021;32(2):263–9.

Economic Considerations of Lung Volume Reduction Surgery and Bronchoscopic Valves

Janani Vigneswaran, MD, MPH[a], Seth Krantz, MD[a,b],*, John Howington, MD[c]

KEYWORDS

• Emphysema • Lung volume reduction surgery • Bronchial valve • QALY • Cost-effective

KEY POINTS

- Chronic obstructive pulmonary disease (COPD) is associated with a substantial burden to the health care system and society, as it relates to direct medical costs and indirect costs.
- In select patients with predominantly upper lobe disease and low exercise tolerance. lung volume reduction surgery can be a cost-effective procedure.
- In select patients without collateral ventilation bronchial valve, therapy can be a cost-effective procedure.
- As surgical and bronchoscopic techniques are refined, length of stay, complication rate. and correct patient selection will improve cost-effectiveness of these lung volume reduction procedures

INTRODUCTION

Chronic obstructive pulmonary disease (COPD) remains a leading cause of chronic morbidity and is the third leading cause of mortality within the United States.[1] For heavy current or former smokers, the prevalence of COPD is approximately 20%, impacting at least 16 million people in the United States.[2] It contributes to a significant reduction in quality of life with substantial economic, societal, and personal costs.

Prevention of COPD exacerbations and the high costs associated with hospital admission remain a major quality goal of the US health care system. For many patients, the disease can be well controlled with medications alone, while for patients with the most severe disease, lung transplant is an effective, although extremely expensive and highly resource-limited option. For patents with significant disease who are not candidates for transplant, treatments focused on reducing dead space and improving ventilation-perfusion matching have shown to be efficacious. This can be done surgically, by resecting the diseased lung, or via 1-way valves that prevent airflow into the diseased area but do allow air to return. These 2 procedures, lung volume reduction surgery (LVRS) and bronchoscopic lung volume reduction (BLVR), have different costs and effectiveness. The economic impacts of these therapies, relative to each other and to best medical practice, is the focus of this article.

CHRONIC OBSTRUCTIVE PULMONARY DISEASE ECONOMIC BURDEN

COPD is associated with a substantial economic burden to the health care system and society as a whole. Understanding the cost of the disease is important for health care decision makers to

[a] Department of Surgery, University of Chicago Medicine & Biological Sciences, Chicago, IL, USA; [b] Division of Thoracic Surgery, Northshore University Health System, Evanston, IL, USA; [c] Department of Clinical Medicine Education, University of Tennessee Health Sciences Center, Ascension Saint Thomas Health, Nashville, TN, USA
* Corresponding author. NorthShore University Health System, 2650 Ridge Avenue, Walgreen Suite 3507, Evanston, IL 60201.
E-mail address: Skrantz@northshore.or.g

Thorac Surg Clin 31 (2021) 211–219
https://doi.org/10.1016/j.thorsurg.2021.02.006
1547-4127/21/© 2021 Elsevier Inc. All rights reserved.

inform policy and guide resource-allocation toward interventions that have the most impact on overall disease-related health care costs and the greatest improvement in patient quality of life. In 2009, US costs attributable to COPD totaled $50 billion, with direct cost estimated at $29.6 billion and indirect costs estimated at $20.4 billion.[3]

Direct costs to the health care system include those related to the detection, treatment, prevention, and rehabilitation of the disease. The direct costs of COPD on the US health care system are substantial. The 2017 Agency for Healthcare Research and Quality group data report total expenditures of COPD at $79 billion, in comparison to cancer at $106 billion, diabetes at $104 billion, and hypertension at $46 billion.[4] COPD consistently ranks among the top 5 most expensive chronic diseases.[5]

Patients with poorly controlled disease have significantly higher costs because of more primary care interactions, more emergency room visits, and increased hospital and intensive care unit admissions.[6] Although total treatment costs are highly correlated with disease severity, within each stage it is still hospitalization expenses that remain the highest portion of costs[7] (see **Table 1** for direct cost breakdown). Targeting interventions that reduce hospitalizations will therefore have the most impact on direct costs.

When considering the economic impact of disease on society, it is also important to understand the indirect costs of the disease. Indirect costs are those costs borne by the patient and society because of the disabling effects of the disease and include loss of productivity, loss of salary, caregiver time and lost productivity, and use of disability benefits. As work productivity and disability benefits are among the largest drivers of indirect costs, the percentage of patients who are working age has a large impact on the societal burden of the disease. In the Confronting COPD in North America and Europe survey, researchers found 82% of COPD patients in the United States are of working age.[8] Patients of working age were asked how often their COPD affected their capacity to work. The results found a dramatic impact on productivity, with over 50% of the population reporting that the disease affected their work productivity. Thirty-five percent of respondents were completely prevented from working during the previous year; 18% were limited in the work they were able to do, and an additional 5% had absences from work. The Health and Retirement Study evaluated the impact of the COPD on Americans older than 50 years with regards to employment status and the collection of disability benefits.[9] These researchers found having COPD resulted in a 9% decrease in likelihood of being employed, a 3.9% increase in probability of collecting Social Security Disability Insurance (SSDI), and a 1.7% increase in likelihood of collecting Supplemental Security Income (SSI). This negative impact on employment exceeds nearly all other major chronic health conditions including heart disease, cancer, hypertension, and diabetes. Only stroke patients experience a comparable decline in employment productivity. Moreover, the associations of COPD with collecting SSDI and SSI are the largest of any of the chronic disease conditions evaluated. At the time of this study, the average wage loss was $38,844, SSDI average annual benefit $14,507, and SSI average annual benefit $6008, for a total societal economic loss of nearly $60,000 per patient. Further compounding the issue is that these are almost certainly underestimates of the broader societal and patient impact, as many indirect costs are difficult to capture. In many cost-effectiveness studies, these costs described previously, as well as costs of out-of-pocket expenses such as nonprescription medication, travel costs to and from health care visits, economic value of the care provided by family members, and time spent by the patient receiving treatment, are not included. Overall, this may lead to potential underestimation of the total economic burden.

Table 1
Direct costs (costs in Canadian dollars, 2004)

	Price
Intensive care unit (ICU) stay	$1446/d
Non-ICU stay	$626/d
General practitioner visit	$54/visit
Emergency room visit	$123/visit
Specialist visit	Varies
Oxygen	$383/month
Medications	$1175
Rehabilitation	$56/outpatient
Mean hospitalization for exacerbation (in the United States)	$18,120[36]

Adapted from Miller JD, Malthaner RA, Goldsmith CH, et al. A randomized clinical trial of lung volume reduction surgery versus best medical care for patients with advanced emphysema: a two-year study From Canada. *Ann Thorac Surg* 2006;81(1):314-321; with permission; Additional data from AbuDagga A, Sun SX, Tan H, Solem CT. Exacerbations among chronic bronchitis patients treated with maintenance medications from a US managed care population: an administrative claims data analysis. *Int J Chron Obstruct Pulmon Dis*. 2013;8:175-185.

HISTORY OF LUNG VOLUME REDUCTION SURGERY AND COSTS

LVRS was first described in 1957, when Brantigan and colleagues[10,11] reported their initial results with multiple wedge resections of emphysematous lung. The procedure showed promise of significant functional improvement, but was abandoned due to perioperative mortality that approached 20%. In 1995 and 1996, Cooper and colleagues reported their results, demonstrating an initial 82% improvement in forced expiratory volume in 1 second (FEV1) with significant symptomatic improvement, with a 90-day mortality of only 4%.[12] Despite these promising results, in 1995, Medicare made the decision not to reimburse LVRS.

The denial of coverage in light of the promising data from Cooper and colleagues is what ultimately led to the National Emphysema Treatment Trial (NETT). This trial confirmed a significant improvement in quality of life and survival for certain subgroups undergoing LVRS, while also identifying patients for whom the procedure was harmful.[13] For non-high-risk patients, there was an improvement in survival, exercise capacity, and quality of life, with the greatest benefit seen in those patients with upper lobe predominant disease and low exercise capacity. As a result of the NETT data, LVRS achieved limited approval by the Centers for Medicare and Medicaid Services (CMS) for select hospital programs and specific patient populations.

Cost-Effectiveness

As part of the NETT report, a companion study evaluating cost-effectiveness was performed. The study included both the direct costs, specifically surgical costs, hospital days, and medications, along with indirect costs such as transportation and time spent by patients and family members related to the care of their disease. **Table 2** shows the breakdown of costs of LVRS compared with best medical care. The study found that after excluding the highest risk patients, who were unlikely to benefit from surgery, the incremental cost-effectiveness ratio (ICER) for LVRS was $190,000 per quality-adjusted life year gained (QALY).[14] With statistical modeling to 10 years, the ratio decreased to $53,000 per QALY gained. The patients with upper lobe predominant disease with low exercise capacity had overall greatest improvement in survival and quality of life, with projected 10-year cost of $21,000 per QALY gained.

In 2006, the data from the multicenter Canadian randomized controlled trial comparing LVRS versus best medical care were published.[15] The researchers found that the LVRS group had a 0.21 improvement in QALY compared with best medical care, and the cost difference was $28,119. For the 2-year study period data, ICER was $133,900 per QALY gained.

Drivers of Cost-Effectiveness

Although the authors from the NETT group looked at direct and indirect costs, it was the direct cost that overwhelmingly drove the cost of care, and of direct costs, number of hospitalization days was the single largest cost driver.[14] The surgery group has 23.3 days in the hospital in the first 6 months, compared with 3 days for the medical group, with an associated total direct medical cost per patient in the surgery group of $62,753 in the first 12 months, compared with $12,932 over the first year per patient in the medical group. These numbers reversed in year 2, with the medical group having higher costs and more hospital days. Further reducing perioperative morbidity and postsurgical length of stay could thus improve the cost-effectiveness ratio for surgery patients, especially the upper lobe-predominant, lower exercise capacity group.

Surgical Approach and Cost

Among the NETT surgical patients, both median sternotomy and video-assisted thoracoscopic surgery (VATS) approaches were utilized; although sternotomy was the dominant approach (359 sternotomy vs 152 VATS). In a nonrandomized comparison of these 2 cohorts, there was no difference in perioperative morbidity or mortality, but there was a shorter length of stay, earlier return to independent living, and overall lower cost for the VATS group.[16] As hospitalization is the largest cost, understanding the main determinants of length of stay is key to reducing the costs associated with LVRS. Although the largest driver of length of stay (LOS) in both groups was air leaks, the rates of air leak at 7 days between the 2 groups were similar (46% sternotomy vs 49% VATS). In a randomized cohort comparing the groups, VATS patients had a median LOS of 6 fewer days than sternotomy patients (9 days vs 15 days). Finally, within the randomized cohort, total cost for VATS was $6500 less per patient over the first 6 months compared with sternotomy.

Improvement in Long-Term Outcomes

Apart from lowering costs, improvements in effectiveness also significantly impact the cost-effectiveness ratio. The NETT follow-up was a median of 2.4 years,[13,17] and the long-term

Table 2
Costs of lung volume reduction surgery (data adjusted to 2020 US dollars)

		Lung Volume Reduction Surgery	Best Medical Care
	Surgery (including bronchoscopy and tracheostomy)	$4882	$0
Index hospitalization	Length of stay	30,248	0
	Total index hospitalization	35,130	0
2 y of follow up costs	Hospitalizations	7509	12,670
	Rehabilitation	3616	2759
	Oxygen	2899	4125
	Medications	1225	1459
	Outpatient visits	1589	1561
	Total follow-up costs	16, 838	22,574
Total Costs		$51, 968	$22,574

Adapted from Miller JD, Malthaner RA, Goldsmith CH, et al. A randomized clinical trial of lung volume reduction surgery versus best medical care for patients with advanced emphysema: a two-year study From Canada. *Ann Thorac Surg* 2006;81(1):314-321; with permission.

projections assumed that the differences in outcomes persisted to 3 years. However, in 2006, a long-term analysis of the outcomes found that the benefits persisted for up to 5 years.[17] Excluding high-risk patients, there was an 18% relative risk reduction of death for LVRS patients at 5 years, and 15% of LVRS patients had a clinically significant improvement in quality of life at 5 years compared with only 7% of medical patients.[17] Among upper lobe-predominant, low-exercise participants, there was a 43% reduction in mortality at 5 years, while 19% had a clinically significant quality-of-life improvements, compared with 0% of the medically treated patients. For the upper lobe-predominant high exercise capacity subgroup, there was a significant palliative benefit, with 23% of LVRS patients having significant quality-of-life improvements persisting to 5 years, compared with only 13% of the medical subgroup.

Utilizing an additional 2 years of data, Ramsey and colleagues performed an updated cost-effectiveness analysis to NETT cost analysis.[18] They found that the 5-year cost for LVRS patients compared with medical patients was $140,000 per QALY gained, which compared favorably with the $190,000 per QALY based on observed 3-year data. For the upper-lobe, low exercise capacity group, the ratio improved from $98,000 per QALY to $77,000 per QALY gained. The other groups also showed improved ICERs. See details in **Table 3**.

HISTORY OF ENDOBRONCHIAL THERAPY AND COSTS

BLVR refers to several different non-surgical interventional techniques for treating severe emphysema. The first and most widely used is the bronchial valve, which is designed to allow 1-way airflow through the airways. The clinical applicability and use of bronchoscopic valves for COPD began in 2007 with publication of a small multi-center study with 30 patients utilizing the Spiration valve, which showed significant improvement in patient-reported quality of life.[19] In 2010, the Emphysema Palliation (VENT) Trial[20] evaluated efficacy of the Zephyr valve placement and showed significant clinical improvement, with the most dramatic improvements seen in patients with a complete fissure. Three subsequent trials, STELVIO, TRANSFORM, and LIBERATE, showed similar clinical improvements with placement of EBV.[21–23] The IMPACT trial evaluated Zephyr valve placement in patients with homogenous emphysema without collateral ventilation, which again showed clinical improvement, but demonstrated that the primary determinant of clinical benefit from EBV is the absence of collateral ventilation, rather than the pattern of emphysema.[24] In June 2018, the US Food and Drug Administration (FDA) approved the Zephyr endobronchial valves as the first bronchoscopic treatment for emphysema in the United States.[25]

Following the success of the Zephyr trials, The REACH and EMPROVE trials re-evaluated the Spiration valve on a larger scale and found statistically significant improvements in clinical markers of lung function.[26,27] In December 2018, the FDA approved the Spiration IBV for treatment of emphysema.[28] In December 2018, the National Institute for Health Care Excellence in the United Kingdom followed suit to recommend the use of bronchial valves for use in emphysema patients.[29]

Table 3
Projected and observed cost-effectiveness ratios for LVRS vs maximal medical therapy for observed and projected years of follow-up from initial randomization, using observations up to 3 years and 5 years after randomization

Incremental Cost-Effectiveness Ratio	All Patients	Upper Lobe Emphysema, Low Exercise Capacity	Upper Lobe Emphysema, High Exercise Capacity	Non-upper Lobe Emphysema, Low Exercise Capacity
Observed up to 3 y	$190,000	$98,000	$240,000	$330,000
Observed up to 5 y	140,000	77,000	170,000	225,000
Projected at 10 y based on 3 y of follow-up	58,000	21,000	54,000	Dominant
Projected at 10 y based on 5 y of follow up	$54,000	$48,000	$40,000	$87,000

From Ramsey SD, Shroyer AL, Sullivan SD, Wood DE. Updated Evaluation of the Cost-effectiveness of Lung Volume Reduction Surgery. *CHEST* 2007;131(3):823-832; with permission.

Shortly thereafter, the 2019 GOLD Report detailed guidelines for the appropriate use of broncho-scopic interventions in select patients with advanced emphysema.[30]

Cost-Effectiveness

Cost analyses for the valves have been performed utilizing data from the original VENT and STELVIO trials. Within the VENT study, researchers evaluated the subgroup of patients who met the current clinical recommendations for bronchial valve therapy: emphysema diagnosis with high heterogeneity, complete fissures isolating the target lobe, and lobar exclusion. They captured direct medical costs obtained from 2014 German Diagnosis Related Group (G-DRG) reimbursement rates.[31] The analysis incorporated procedure costs (assuming an average of 3 valves per procedure) and included all clinical events during the 12-month follow-up with Markov modeling used to project costs for years 2 to 10. They found in the 5-year model, EBV costs were $30,313 versus control $15,256, and QALY in the EBV group was 2.88 versus control 2.66. The calculated ICERs were $67,722 and $36,757 per QALY gained for the 5 year and 10-year models, respectively[a]. In a separate study, data from the STELVIO trial were used to calculate direct medical costs from the hospital perspective, derived from Dutch health insurance price levels in 2016.[32] The analysis included an expected 5-day LOS, assumed average of 4.5 valves per procedure, and included all clinical events within the first 6 months, with a Markov simulation model to determine long-term economic value at 5 and 10 years. The authors found with a 5-year modeling analysis a cost of $46,937 per QALY gained and for 10-year modeling a cost of $25,876 per QALY gained[b].

Drivers of Cost-Effectiveness

Hartman and colleagues[33] reviewed the breakdown of costs in the valve group compared with the control group. Most of the total costs that came from the EBV group were from the initial bronchoscopy and the associated products used. Furthermore, in the instance in which there was a complication that required intervention with repeat bronchoscopy (35%), there was an even larger expense associated with the total cost. In this study, with just 6 months of follow-up data, there did not appear to be a huge difference in the COPD exacerbation rates among the control group and EBV group, which is a large limitation in the study, because as was seen in the NETTs trial, the benefit of intervention was most seen in the second year after the procedure.[14] Longer-term follow-up with data of both the control group and the EBV group would likely lead to larger differences for COPD-specific complications from standard medical therapy compared with EBV placement. Also, with provider experience in use of placement of EBVs, it is likely the complication rates will decrease, thus, further improving the cost-effectiveness ratio for EBV patients.

---

[a]Costs reported here are converted from 2014 Euros to the 2020 US dollar.

[b]Costs reported here are converted from 2016 Euros to the 2020 US dollar.

Table 4
Variation in cost analysis among studies (data adjusted to 2020 US dollars)

Study	Years of Data	Cost per QALY Gained
US NETT 2003[16]	3 y	$272,270
US NETT 2003[16] (subgroup with most clinical benefit: upper lobe emphysema, with low exercise capacity)	3 y	140,434
Canadian RCT 2006[9]	2 y	134,365
Ramsey et al,[18] 2007 NETT update	5 y	196,149
Ramsey et al,[18] 2007 NETT update (subgroup with most clinical benefit: upper lobe emphysema, with low exercise capacity)	5 y	107,822
German EBV Study[19] modeling projections for 5 y	12 months	69,611
Dutch EBV Study[20] modeling projections for 5 y	6 months	$46,498

Data from Refs.[14,15,20,32,33]

COST-EFFECTIVENESS COMPARISON OF LUNG VOLUME REDUCTION SURGERY AND ENDOBRONCHIAL VALVES

Within a health care system with limited budgets, it is important for medical care payers to determine the value of each novel therapy, as each approved reimbursement of a new cost increasing technology could potentially displace payments for other areas of health care. In the instance of LVRS versus BLVR, it also ensures that therapies are applied to the most suitable patients, as the clinical outcomes vary largely depending on the type of emphysema. In selecting COPD patients who are most likely to benefit from LVRS, data would suggest that those with predominantly upper-lobe emphysema and low exercise capacity have the greatest improvement in terms of survival and functional outcomes compared with medical therapy. Conversely, the optimal COPD patient to benefit from a valve placement is one with a complete fissure and thus no collateral ventilation to the lobe that the provider is aiming to occlude. An important difference from LVRS is that the bronchial valve clinical trials demonstrated equal clinical effectiveness in both upper and lower lobe-predominant emphysema.[33]

A direct comparison of the ICERs for LVRS and BLVR is challenging. The data were collected from different time periods and in different health care systems. The LVRS data are from early 1997 to 2003, from US and Canadian health care systems, while the BLVR cost analysis was done from 2014

to 2016 in European health care systems. Table 4 includes costs adjusted to US dollars and accounted for inflation to demonstrate anticipated cost per QALY gained in 2020. Additionally, because bronchial valve placement therapy for COPD is a relatively new technique, there has been no true 5- and 10-year cost analysis follow-up done, only projections based on assumed efficacy. As the data from LVRS demonstrated, 5- and 10-year modeling can be dramatically different from the true long-term outcomes (see **Table 4**).[18] As of now, however, the data would suggest the clinical benefit of EBV therapy lasts for at least a 5-year follow-up.[34] Perhaps most challenging is the changing nature of the costs of a given procedure. As discussed previously, most of the LVRS patients in the analysis had a median sternotomy; however, the current preferred surgical approach is VATS, which is associated with lower overall costs than sternotomy.[16] Similarly, as providers become more comfortable with the bronchoscopic technique, it is likely that the complication rates and LOS will improve and, subsequently, costs will decrease. Finally, the LVRS studies were done before implementation of various national quality improvement programs that have led to great improvements in health care quality indicators, including lower rates of reintubation and prolonged ventilation.

FUTURE MEDICAL COSTS

Akuthota and colleagues[35] performed an analysis from their pulmonary function test laboratory database from 1996 to 2006 searching patients with GOLD III and IV COPD. They estimated up to 15% of the general population of advanced emphysema patients are potential candidates for LVRS.

However, the limited number of CMS-approved sites for performing LVRS and hesitation on the side of patients and referring providers has limited the number of procedures to less than 1000 per year in the United States. In a review of the STS Database from January 2003 to June 2011, Decker and colleagues[35] noted only 538 patients underwent LVRS in 8.5 years, with a high of 118 cases in 2008. Future growth in treatment of patients with advanced (GOLD III and IV) emphysema will likely be in treatment with BLVR. This endoscopic approach is not limited to the CMS-approved sites for LVRS. Data from the VENT trial would suggest that 37% of patients with advanced emphysema had complete fissures eligible for treatment.

Based on US Centers for Disease Control and Prevention (CDC) and severity data, it is estimated there are 1.5 million severe emphysema patients in the United States. Of these, 80% are predicted to have sufficient hyperinflation for volume reduction. Of these, another 20% would be ineligible for treatment because of comorbidities, lung destruction, or lung morphology. Another 50% would be ineligible due to collateral ventilation. Thus, approximately 500,000 patients would be eligible for treatment with BLVR. The advanced emphysema population is growing by 1% to 2% a year, and the average life expectancy for these patients is about 10 years, meaning approximately 10% to 12% of the prevalent base is comprised of patients newly diagnosed with severe emphysema each year.

The biggest challenge in predicting future cost is that most of these patients are not currently referred for treatment, and many are not under the care of a pulmonologist. Ideally, patients would be sent to a center offering pulmonary rehabilitation, surgery, and bronchial valves for workup that included radiological, nuclear medicine, blood gas, exercise and pulmonary function assessments, and personalized care recommendations. Because BLVR was only recently approved by the FDA and similar international bodies, it will take many years to begin making the necessary changes to referral patterns to get patients to routinely be referred to COPD centers of excellence.

SUMMARY

Prevention of COPD exacerbations and hospitalizations remains a major quality goal for health care systems. In patients with severe emphysema-related COPD, hospitalizations remain the primary driver of the high cost of care. In the United States,

it is estimated that the total societal economic loss associated with COPD is nearly $60,000 per year. In properly selected patient cohorts, both LVRS and BLVR have proven cost-effective.

The data show LVRS has the greatest clinical benefit and cost-effectiveness in patients with upper lobe predominant emphysema and low exercise tolerance. In addition, this cohort had the lowest 30-day mortality rate, at 2.9% in the NETT trial.[36] LVRS remains clinically effective and reduces costs in patients with upper lobe-predominant emphysema and high exercise capacity. Recent trials show BLVR is clinically effective and cost-effective in emphysema patients with low exercise capacity and complete fissures irrespective of whether the disease is upper lobe predominant or homogenous.

At first pass, one could conclude that homogenous patients should be approached with BLVR and upper lobe predominant patients approached with minimally invasive (VATS) LVRS. The ICER for upper lobe predominant emphysema patients with low exercise capacity observed for 5 years and projected for 10 years was $48,000 compared with an ICER of $87,000 in non-upper-lobe predominant emphysema patients with low exercise capacity.

A challenge arises in trying to effectively identify patients with a complete fissure. Each trial showed an approximate 20% incidence of collateral ventilation based on bronchoscopic investigation of patients with HRCT examinations, suggesting complete fissures. The need to cross-over these 20% of patients to evaluation for LVRS will add to the overall cost of care. An encouraging finding in the studies was the retained eligibility for surgical LVRS in patients requiring removal of the endobronchial valves.

The less-invasive nature of BLVR and the embracement of the technology by pulmonary medicine physicians will hopefully increase referrals of advanced emphysema patients for lung volume reduction at multidisciplinary centers.

CLINICS CARE POINTS

- Upper lobe-predominant emphysema patients with low exercise capacity after formal pulmonary rehabilitation should be managed with bilateral VATS LVRS.

- Non-upper lobe emphysema patients without collateral ventilation should be managed with BLVR.

- Any procedure performed on a cohort of patients at higher risk for complications and

> poor tolerance of adverse outcomes requires a multidisciplinary approach to optimal patient selection.
> - Proper patient selection and periprocedural patient management play a more significant role in outcomes for this patient population than nuances of procedural technique.

DISCLOSURE

The authors report nothing to disclose.

REFERENCES

1. Health, United States. 2016 with Chartbook on Long-Term Trends in Health. U.S. Department of Health and Human Service; Centers for Disease Control and Prevention; National Center for Health Statistics; 2017. Available at: https://www.cdc.gov/nchs/data/hus/hus16.pdf. Accessed July 3, 2020.
2. Wheaton AG. Chronic obstructive pulmonary disease and smoking status — United States, 2017. MMWR Morb Mortal Wkly Rep 2019;68:533–8.
3. Morbidity & mortality: 2012 chart book on cardiovascular, lung, and blood diseases. p. 117.
4. MEPS summary tables. Available at: https://meps.ahrq.gov/mepstrends/hc_cond_icd10/. Accessed July 3, 2020.
5. Soni A. Statistical BRIEF #470: trends in the five most costly conditions among the U.S. civilian noninstitutionalized population, 2002 and 2012. Available at: https://meps.ahrq.gov/data_files/publications/st470/stat470.shtml. Accessed July 25, 2020.
6. Iheanacho I, Zhang S, King D, et al. Economic burden of chronic obstructive pulmonary disease (COPD): a systematic literature review. Int J Chronic Obstructive Pulm Dis 2020;15:439–60.
7. Hilleman DE, Dewan N, Malesker M, et al. Pharmacoeconomic evaluation of COPD. Chest 2000; 118(5):1278–85.
9. Thornton Snider J, Romley JA, Wong KS, et al. The disability burden of COPD. COPD J Chronic Obstr Pulm Dis 2012;9(5):513–21.
8. Wouters EFM. Economic analysis of the confronting COPD survey: an overview of results. Respir Med 2003;97(Suppl C):S3–14.
10. Brantigan OC, Mueller E. Surgical treatment of pulmonary emphysema. Am Surg 1957;23(9):789–804.
11. Brantigan OC, Mueller E, Kress MB. A surgical approach to pulmonary emphysema. Am Rev Respir Dis 1959;80(1 Part 2):194–206.
12. Cooper JD, Patterson GA, Sundaresan RS, et al. Results of 150 consecutive bilateral lung volume reduction procedures in patients with severe emphysema. J Thorac Cardiovasc Surg 1996;112(5):1319–29 [discussion 1329-1330].
13. Criner GJ, Sternberg AL. National emphysema treatment trial. Proc Am Thorac Soc 2008;5(4):393–405.
14. Cost effectiveness of lung-volume–reduction surgery for patients with severe emphysema. N Engl J Med 2003;348(21):2092–102.
15. Miller JD, Malthaner RA, Goldsmith CH, et al. A randomized clinical trial of lung volume reduction surgery versus best medical care for patients with advanced emphysema: a two-year study from Canada. Ann Thorac Surg 2006;81(1):314–21.
16. McKenna RJ, Benditt JO, DeCamp M, et al. Safety and efficacy of median sternotomy versus video-assisted thoracic surgery for lung volume reduction surgery. J Thorac Cardiovasc Surg 2004;127(5):1350–60.
17. Naunheim KS, Wood DE, Mohsenifar Z, et al. Long-term follow-up of patients receiving lung-volume-reduction surgery versus medical therapy for severe emphysema by the National Emphysema Treatment Trial Research Group. Ann Thorac Surg 2006;82(2):431–43.
18. Ramsey SD, Shroyer AL, Sullivan SD, et al. Updated evaluation of the cost-effectiveness of lung volume reduction surgery. Chest 2007;131(3):823–32.
19. Wood DE, McKenna RJ, Yusen RD, et al. A multicenter trial of an intrabronchial valve for treatment of severe emphysema. J Thorac Cardiovasc Surg 2007;133(1):65–73.e2.
20. Sciurba FC, Ernst A, Herth FJF, et al. A randomized study of endobronchial valves for advanced emphysema. N Engl J Med 2010;363(13):1233–44.
21. Klooster K, Hartman JE, ten Hacken NHT, et al. One-year follow-up after endobronchial valve treatment in patients with emphysema without collateral ventilation treated in the STELVIO trial. Respiration 2017; 93(2):112–21.
22. Kemp SV, Slebos D-J, Kirk A, et al. A multicenter randomized controlled trial of zephyr endobronchial valve treatment in heterogeneous emphysema (TRANSFORM). Am J Respir Crit Care Med 2017; 196(12):1535–43.
23. Criner GJ, Sue R, Wright S, et al. A multicenter randomized controlled trial of zephyr endobronchial valve treatment in heterogeneous emphysema (LIBERATE). Am J Respir Crit Care Med 2018; 198(9):1151–64.
24. Valipour A, Slebos D-J, Herth F, et al. Endobronchial valve therapy in patients with homogeneous emphysema. results from the IMPACT study. Am J Respir Crit Care Med 2016;194(9):1073–82.
25. Health C for D and R. Zephyr® Endobronchial Valve System - P180002. FDA. Published online February 9, 2019. Available at: https://www.fda.gov/medical-devices/recently-approved-devices/zephyrr-

endobronchial-valve-system-p180002. Accessed July 24, 2020.

29. Endobronchial valve Insertion to reduce lung volume in emphysema. National Institute for Health Care Excellence; 2017. Available at: https://www.nice.org.uk/guidance/ipg600/resources/endobronchial-valve-insertion-to-reduce-lung-volume-in-emphysema-pdf-1899873854992069.

26. Li S, Wang G, Wang C, et al. The REACH trial: a randomized controlled trial assessing the safety and effectiveness of the Spiration® valve system in the treatment of severe emphysema. Respiration 2019; 97(5):416–27.

27. Criner GJ, Delage A, Voelker K, et al. Improving lung function in severe heterogenous emphysema with the Spiration valve system (EMPROVE). a multicenter, open-label randomized controlled clinical trial. Am J Respir Crit Care Med 2019;200(11): 1354–62.

28. Health C for D and R. Spiration Valve® system - P180007. FDA; 2019. Available at: https://www.fda.gov/medical-devices/recently-approved-devices/spiration-valver-system-p180007. Accessed July 24, 2020.

30. Global strategy for the diagnosis, management, and prevention of chronic obstructive pulmonary disease (2019 Report). Global Initiative for chronic obstructive lung disease. Available at: https://goldcopd.org/wp-content/uploads/2018/11/GOLD-2019-v1.7-FINAL-14Nov2018-WMS.pdf. Accessed July 24, 2020.

31. Pietzsch JB, Garner A, Herth FJF. Cost-effectiveness of endobronchial valve therapy for severe emphysema: a model-based projection based on the VENT study. Respiration 2014;88(5):389–98.

32. Hartman JE, Klooster K, Groen H, et al. Cost-effectiveness of endobronchial valve treatment in patients with severe emphysema compared to standard medical care: cost-effectiveness of EBV treatment. Respirology 2018;23(9):835–41.

33. Valipour A. Valve therapy in patients with emphysematous type of chronic obstructive pulmonary disease (COPD): from randomized trials to patient selection in clinical practice. J Thorac Dis 2018; 10(Suppl 23):S2780–96.

34. Garner J, Kemp SV, Toma TP, et al. Survival after endobronchial valve placement for emphysema: a 10-year follow-up study. Am J Respir Crit Care Med 2016;194(4):519–21.

35. Akuthota P, Litmanovich D, Zutler M, et al. An evidence-based estimate on the size of the potential patient pool for lung volume reduction surgery. Ann Thorac Surg 2012;94(1):205–11.

36. Decker MR, Leverson GE, Jaoude WA, et al. Lung volume reduction surgery since the National Emphysema Treatment Trial: study of society of thoracic surgeons database. J Thorac Cardiovasc Surg 2014;148(6):2651–8.e1.

Future Treatment of Emphysema with Roles for Valves, Novel Strategies and Lung Volume Reduction Surgery

Simran Randhawa, MD, Bryan Meyers, MD, MPH*

KEYWORDS

- Emphysema • Lung volume reduction • Bronchoscopic intervention

KEY POINTS

- Endobronchial valves are the main non-surgical intervention available to address the symptoms of emphysema.
- Multiple alternative strategies have been devised but have failed to achieve the reliable benefits seen with valves.
- Meticulous patient selection and transparent education of risks and benefits will allow the best allocation of surgery and non-surgical alternatives.

Previous articles in this issue chronicle the evolution of surgical attempts to improve lung function and to enhance the quality of life in emphysema patients by reducing the size of emphysematous lungs. The size reduction improves the air flow in the remaining lungs and enhances the matching of ventilation and pulmonary perfusion in the remaining lung tissue. The lineage of interventions actually began in the 1950s with the initial efforts of Otto Brantigan[1] and is punctuated by the pioneering resuscitation of the notion of volume reduction by Cooper and colleagues[2] in 1995.

Along the way, there have been some novel strategies with similar short-term (shrink the lungs) and long-term (improve lung function and reduce dyspnea) goals. Wakabayashi and colleagues reported in 1991 their efforts to treat emphysema by heating and shrinking lung tissue afflicted with bullous emphysema by applying a low-energy CO_2 laser to the surface of the diseased lung tissue. Their initial report[3] showed a nearly 10% mortality rate but

also proved the underlying physiologic principle by demonstrating decreased total lung capacity (volume reduction) and the association with increased forced expiratory volume in 1 second (FEV1) and forced vital capacity (FVC) demonstrated with pre- and postintervention testing.

Although there are multiple pharmacologic and nonpharmacological options to alleviate symptoms, none of these treatment modalities halts disease progression. The expanding disease burden has led to development of innovative therapeutic strategies that also aim to induce lung volume reduction over the past decades. Bronchoscopic lung volume reduction originated in 2001 and has continued to grow rapidly ever since. The previous articles in this issue have discussed lung volume reduction and the use of endobronchial valves for management of emphysema. This article discusses more recent developments in bronchoscopic and novel interventions and speculates on how these novel

Washington University School of Medicine, Barnes-Jewish Hospital, Campus Box 8234, 660 South Euclid Avenue, Saint Louis, MO 63110-1093, USA
* Corresponding author.
E-mail address: meyersb@wustl.edu

Thorac Surg Clin 31 (2021) 221–227
https://doi.org/10.1016/j.thorsurg.2021.02.003
1547-4127/21/© 2021 Elsevier Inc. All rights reserved.

strategies may impact the future of lung reduction interventions.

ENDOBRONCHIAL VALVES

This intervention is covered elsewhere in this issue but deserves brief mention here for the sake of completeness. This is the current mainstay of endoscopic options and therefore seems to be the most likely of any of these alternatives to surgery to be offered. In a recent review of the specialty on interventional pulmonology, Wahidi and colleagues[4] summarized the state of the art in all areas of this evolving subspecialty. Endobronchial valve therapy was the only modality mentioned among the multitude of endoscopic emphysema interventions. The physiologic and symptom improvements seen in trials tracking measured lung function, exercise tolerance, and self-reported quality of life were cited, as were the risks of procedural pneumothorax and uncertainty of the magnitude and duration of benefit for any individual. Valves are the current kingpin of nonsurgical interventions.

LUNG VOLUME REDUCTION COILS

Nitinol coils are shape-memory devices that assume their preformed shape once bronchoscopically deployed into the subsegmental airways. Placed into an airway of some diseased and hyperexpanded lung, the device resumes the coiled shape and pulls the lung tissue into a compressed form, thus reducing the volume. Once they assume their initial and preferred shape, nitinol coils act by compressing the surrounding emphysematous lung parenchyma. In theory, this creates tissue tension and restores radial support to airways, thereby tethering nearby airways open to reduce airway collapse and air trapping during exhalation and exercise. These are nonobstructive devices, and they exert the desired effect immediately, unimpeded by the presence of any collateral ventilation. Since the first publication of endobronchial coil implantation by Herth and colleagues[5] in 2010, much has been published regarding the use of coils as a mode of bronchoscopic lung volume reduction.

Apart from improving the ventilatory mechanics of the affected emphysematous lung, lung reduction coils also potentially increase perfusion adjacent to the treated areas. In a quantitative analysis, Lador and colleagues[6] revealed that coil lung reduction resulted in a significant increase in perfusion to the coil-free areas immediately adjacent to the treated region, as well as in other ipsilateral untreated areas. This redistribution of pulmonary blood flow toward the better ventilated areas was presumed to be the result of better closure of vessels in diseased regions after coil placement, resulting in increased resistance to blood flow in the emphysematous lung and redirection to healthier regions of lower resistance. As a consequence, coil reduction may thus improve the pulmonary ventilation/perfusion ratio.

There have been 3 randomized controlled studies comparing coil lung reduction with medical therapy. The RENEW trial randomly assigned 315 emphysema patients to either a coil treatment group or to a standard medical care group.[7] At 1 year of follow-up, data showed a statistically significant improvement in the 6-min walk distance by 10.3 m with coil treatment ($P=.02$), along with median change in FEV1 by 7% ($P<.001$) and in the St. George's Respiratory Questionnaire with a shift of 8.9 points ($P<.001$), each difference favoring the coil group. The Réduction Volumique Endobronchique par Spirales (REVOLENS) study was a multicenter 1:1 randomized superiority trial comparing coil treatment with a usual care control group in 100 patients.[8] During the 1-year follow-up, authors demonstrated an improvement in exercise capacity with a significant decrease in lung hyperinflation and an associated improvement in self-reported quality of life. Subsequently, the 2 year prospective follow-up study showed sustained improvement in quality of life and a sustained decrease in pulmonary residual volume, with no late-onset events.[9] The longest follow-up study recently completed, the RESET study, showed a survival advantage at 5 years for endobronchial coil implantation in the subset of patients who had achieved a 10% reduction in residual volume (RV) at 3 months.[10] The ELEVATE study is a prospective, multicenter, randomized, controlled study that is currently being conducted to further identify disease characteristics using quantitative computed tomography (CT) scans to determine which patients will respond to coil treatment.[11]

In an attempt to compare outcomes across treatment modalities, Marchetti and colleagues[12] evaluated individuals who received bilateral coil therapy in previously reported trials and compared them with individuals who underwent lung volume reduction surgery (LVRS) within National Emphysema Treatment Trial. They demonstrated that placement of endobronchial coils in patients with advanced homogeneous emphysema reduced residual volume and total lung capacity, and increased walking distance compared with optimal medical therapy. Additionally, their study also showed improved walking distance and survival with coil use when compared with LVRS.

One of the most common complications reported after EBC is pneumonia or lower respiratory tract infections (20% incidence in the REVOLENS trial, 15% incidence in the RENEW trial). However, several of these pneumonias appeared to be noninfectious in nature and are considered by some experts to be secondary to the force of the coils on the lung tissue causing an inflammatory response. This response results in radiographic findings of dense consolidations that are unique to this treatment modality. These so-called coil-associated opacities (CAOs) are difficult to distinguish from pneumonia, and the clinical significance is unknown. Yet another potential drawback with these devices is that they are deemed permanent or at least very difficult to remove. Despite the concern and caveat of permanence, there are isolated reports of successful removal of coils even after 1 year postimplantation.[13]

An expert recommendation panel from 2017 summarized optimal criteria for coil implantation as follows: FEV1 less than 50%, RV less than 175%, RV/total lung capacity (TLC) less than 0.58, 6-minute walk distance 150 to 450 m.[14] They also emphasized on the importance of careful selection of patients, along with routine culture of bronchial secretions during the bronchoscopy procedure, thus addressing the concerns of a high risk for respiratory infections. Frequently, pharmacologic and nonpharmacological treatment need to be optimized before starting a coil treatment. This is crucial given the complexity, expense, and irreversibility of the treatment. Deployment of coils requires a multidisciplinary team approach with pulmonology, radiology, thoracic surgery, and pulmonary rehabilitation in selecting the most appropriate treatment for an individual patient.

BRONCHOSCOPIC THERMAL VAPOR ABLATION

Bronchoscopic thermal vapor ablation is a fairly new treatment modality first described in 2009 as a novel way to reduce lung volume in the setting of emphysema.[15] The mechanism involves bronchoscopic instillation of heated water (at a temperature of 75°C) into the preselected target emphysematous segments. The resulting heat injury induces a local inflammatory reaction. Steam moves through air-containing spaces, and heat dissipation is related to tissue density, structure, and regional blood flow.[16] The inflammatory reaction promotes fibrosis and shrinkage of the targeted ventilated areas, leading to volume reduction of those poorly perfused lung segments. Because this therapy has no effect on the nontargeted lung tissue, bronchoscopic thermal vapor ablation can be used to manage intralobar heterogenous emphysema, with or without presence of collateral ventilation. Furthermore, it is currently the only mode of lung reduction intervention that leaves no implants in the patient.

The STEP-UP trial in 2016 was the first randomized trial comparing bronchoscopic thermal vapor ablation with standard medical treatment for emphysema.[17] In a 6-month follow-up report, results demonstrated a statistically significant 14.7% difference in FEV1 after bilateral thermal ablation compared with the control group, a 9.7-point reduction in St. George Respiratory Questionnaire (SGRQ), and a residual volume reduction of 302.5 mL.[18] Data obtained at the 12-month follow-up visits showed persistent improvements in FEV1 (9.2%) and SGRQ (8.4 points).

Ideal candidates for bronchoscopic thermal vapor ablation are identified using body plethysmography and CT scans. The favorable patients are characterized by severe hyperinflation (RV ≥175%) and upper lobe-predominant emphysema, with an FEV1 and diffusing capacity for carbon monoxide (DLCO) preferably at least 20% because of safety concerns. The targeted segments are identified as those with the highest disease severity, the highest heterogeneity index (HI), and the highest segmental volume.[19] Bronchoscopic thermal vapor ablation is a nonblocking, irreversible technique. The most common adverse events in the STEP-UP trial were chronic obstructive pulmonary disease (COPD) exacerbations and pneumonia/pneumonitis. Treatment of these complications relies on corticosteroids and antimicrobial therapy according to standard care. Clinical trials are underway to further study the benefits and risks with use of bronchoscopic thermal vapor ablation. Data gathered from such studies will enable continued improvement in patient selection and outcomes of vapor ablation over time.[20]

ADDITIONAL NOVEL STRATEGIES

Targeted lung denervation is a novel potential therapeutic intervention for COPD. Using a bronchoscopically guided catheter-based lung denervation system (Holaira, Inc., Plymouth, Minnesota), radiofrequency energy is applied, and parasympathetic pulmonary nerves surrounding the main bronchi are ablated. This disrupts the autonomic input from the vagus nerve that has been shown to be elevated at baseline in COPD patients.[21,22] Consequently, the decreased bronchomotor tone results in bronchodilation and reduces airway hyperresponsiveness and mucus hypersecretion. The first in-human clinical trial by

Slebos and colleagues[23] in 2015 reported an increase of 11.6% in FEV1, an increase of 6.8 min in submaximal exercise cycle endurance, and a decrease of 11.1 points in SGRQ score. Further impacts of targeted lung denervation potentially include disruption of airway inflammatory mediators and airway remodeling.[24] Although it is not a volume reduction procedure and is not yet routinely used in clinical practice, targeted lung denervation may have synergistic effects when combined with other interventions and pharmacologic agents used for COPD management. Future studies are required to further evaluate its efficacy and safety profile.

Polymeric lung volume reduction involves bronchoscopic application of rapidly polymerizing biologic agents to reduce lung volume by blocking off the most emphysematous areas. Once applied, resorption atelectasis occurs from airway occlusion followed by subsequent airspace inflammation, and then remodeling. This remodeling occurs by way of scarring of lung parenchyma that provides a functional volume reduction. Clinical trials have studied the use of fibrin glue[25] and autologous blood patch,[26] with both showing promising results. The only randomized trial, the ASPIRE study published in 2015, demonstrated the intended positive effects but an unfavorable risk profile with this intervention.[27] The study was halted for business reasons after randomization of 95 out the planned 300 subjects. In this study, 44% of treated patients experienced adverse events requiring hospital admission and additional pharmacotherapy including steroids and antibiotics. The most frequent symptoms were pneumonia, COPD exacerbations, and respiratory failure. If adverse effects of this sort of treatment could be reduced or successfully mitigated, the cost-effectiveness and apparent ease of execution make this strategy an attractive intervention, and further research seems prudent. Currently, however, it appears that other forms of intervention are viewed as more favorable for additional development and testing.

Airway bypass was developed based on the observation that patients with severe emphysema had dilated terminal airway spaces and patent central bronchi, but collapsible midlevel airways that impeded exhalation. Creating a path from the dilated terminal airway to the patent central bronchus (airway bypass) could allow improved exhalation and reduce air trapping, lung distention, and dyspnea. To maintain patency of the bypass, stents were placed within the bypass channel with the aim of releasing trapped air from targeted areas. Paclitaxel-coated stents were used in varying numbers. Preliminary work demonstrated the

proof of the principle; however, clinical studies failed to demonstrate significant functional outcomes.[28] Furthermore, there were long-term concerns for granulation tissue growth, stent occlusion, and stent migration, which occurred commonly. Further development of this novel intervention seems to be on hold.

ONGOING CLINICAL TRIALS

A current trial is looking at lung volume reduction for severe emphysema by stereotactic ablative radiation therapy (ClinicalTrials.gov Identifier: NCT03673176). As commonly seen in stereotactic radiation therapy performed for lung cancer treatment, radiation typically leaves a scar in the area of lung that has been treated. This scarring process results in contraction of surrounding lung parenchyma that is essentially a focal example of lung volume reduction. There are existing data regarding lower risk of morbidity and mortality with stereotactic ablative radiotherapy (SABR) in lung cancer surgery, so it seems a clever pivot to see if the same attributes result in a favorable intervention for emphysema. One drawback is that the scarring process is associated with the density of tissue irradiated, and the most diseased portions of lung in emphysema have low density of tissue. It will be interesting to observe as trials unwrap the potential role of stereotactic radiation, a commonly available treatment that is applied with great precision, as a potential strategy for patients with emphysema but no cancer.

Various combinations of bronchoscopic lung reduction methods are also being evaluated. Lung Volume Reduction in Severe Emphysema Using Bronchoscopic Autologous Blood Instillation in Combination With Intra-bronchial Valves (BLOOD-VALVES) is one such pilot study. (ClinicalTrials.gov identifier: NCT03010449). It seems natural that other combination strategies of novel therapies might be considered in the future.

FUTURE ROLE FOR LUNG REDUCTION INTERVENTIONS

Lung reduction in the broad sense is based on the principle that states that by removing diseased emphysematous lung tissue, one can improve symptoms, respiratory physiology, and possibly survival in a clearly identifiable subgroup of patients with advanced emphysema. Despite that accepted principle, with an estimated 3.8 million patients with emphysema in the United States, it is clear that only a miniscule proportion of these patients end up undergoing lung reduction of any kind. This potential treatment option for palliating life that is based on sound clinical and physiologic principles may be underutilized.

One of the main reasons is the perception regarding the potential survival benefits and risks associated with the surgery. Studies evaluating LVRS may possibly have placed a strong emphasis on survival benefits without similar regard for the value of palliation. In a debilitating and progressive disease such as emphysema, however, palliation without lengthening of life span can be especially rewarding. An example might be the subgroup analyzed in the National Emphysema Treatment Trial (NETT), in which patients had upper lobe predominant emphysema and high exercise tolerance. Those patients did not receive a predictable survival advantage with lung volume reduction surgery, but they did receive a durable advantage in exercise tolerance, relief from respiratory symptoms, and patient-reported quality of life.

Furthermore, in NETT, patients were enrolled between 1998 and 2002. Since then, much progress has been made both in the surgical approach leading to broad adoption of minimally invasive approaches (VATS and robotic) in the surgery, and enhancements in postoperative care. Hence, this fairly rare operation has the potential to be revived with modern surgical technology, much as the original Brantigan operation was revived by Cooper after the passage of 4 decades of incremental improvements in imaging, medications, surgical technology, and perioperative care. In the same period of time, from 1998 to 2021, the authors have seen the expected and acceptable mortality of a lobectomy for lung cancer drop from 3% to 4% to less than 1%. It seems reasonable to think that the same could occur with surgical lung volume reduction.

Careful patient selection remains key, regardless of the technique or approach. This maxim goes back to the 1990s, when Cooper and colleagues released their first series of patients treated with LVRS. They emphasized from their experience that favorable outcomes from LVRS required careful selection of appropriate patients, and multidisciplinary team approach by pulmonologists, thoracic surgeons, and other relevant specialists. The same remains true today with other methods of reducing lung volume to address symptoms of emphysema. In the main result paper from the LIBERATE trial demonstrating efficacy for endobronchial valves, the authors described the fact that 909 patients were consented for evaluation and treatment, but only 160 patients met the full inclusion trial.[29] Just as with the early studies in surgical volume reduction, the sweet spot of appropriate hyperexpansion, location of disease, disease that is severe but not too severe, preserved functional reserve and acceptable comorbid conditions remain elusive challenges.

The challenge that lies ahead is to ensure that all lung volume reduction therapies are individualized, comprehensive, and patient-focused. This will require development of expert centers with multidisciplinary teams and availability of all treatment modalities and surgeon expertise for patient care and further development of lung volume reduction therapies. The notion of personalized medicine is increasingly emphasized in all aspects of the shared medical field and in some notable areas of thoracic surgery. The increased knowledge about targeted therapy, immunotherapy, and mutational analysis of lung cancer has been transformative. The current strategy for matching patients to specific drugs for adjuvant or definitive chemotherapy bears no resemblance to the strategy relied upon 10 years ago. It seems reasonable that the accumulated data from many surgical and bronchoscopic volume reduction clinical trials, in addition to data from administrative databases describing actual care provided in the modern era, could be mined to provide personalized expectations for outcomes for all interventions. This would allow better shared decision making for the patient and enhanced collaboration among the specialists to offer the appropriate intervention.

Transparency of outcomes has done much to improve patient selection and quality improvement processes throughout the surgical field. The knowledge that outcomes from a single institution or even a single practitioner might be available for comparison with outcomes from others has certainly altered behavior in the cardiothoracic surgical field. Surgical mortality used to be viewed as the inevitable risk associated with taking bold steps toward a positive outcome. Surgical databases and public reporting have certainly influenced risk tolerance and the broad consideration of multimodality treatment options. Ongoing monitoring and public reporting of the risk of death and complications, as well as the benefits derived from all of the interventions aimed at emphysema, would provide critical information to patients and those advising them. This type of information should be demanded by specialty insiders, disease advocacy groups, and payors.

New parameters for study have been created using clever utilization of existing technology and analytics that might better inform patient selection for volume reduction intervention. Analytical morphomics is a novel approach using semiautomated image processing to quantitate various aspects of body composition from standard preoperative CT scans. These are objective measurements of physical properties that might be missed by the standard clinician view, but which are highly associated with outcomes when measured and analyzed systematically. For example, Lin and colleagues at the University of Michigan demonstrated that there are numerous, readily available, morphomic factors that are associated with physiologic reserve and frailty and could serve as independent predictors of survival, prolonged ventilation, and excessive length of stay after lung transplantation.[30] The authors suggested that routine use of morphomics preoperatively could improve recipient selection and risk stratification. If such as strategy could be useful for predicting outcomes in lung transplantation, it certainly could offer important insights when considering treatment options for lung volume reduction intervention.

It seems unlikely that any single modality will emerge as a dominant therapy in this highly nuanced field. However, with meticulous patient selection to identify and include those most likely to benefit and to identify and exclude those most likely to suffer treatment related complications, one can make the best case for specific intervention above and beyond best medical therapy. One size most assuredly does not fit all in this particular arena. One patient might agree to a 3% to 4% mortality risk in order to get a 25% to 40% increase in pulmonary function, whereas other patients might prefer a 1% mortality risk to achieve a 10% to 15% increase in pulmonary function. Additionally, optimal patient preparation with minimally invasive surgical intervention and expert perioperative recovery can provide the interventional boost intended by the chosen therapy while minimizing the potential associated complications.

CLINICS CARE POINTS

- Lung volume reductions ought to be individualized and patient focused, and require a multi-disciplinary team approach comprising experts in surgical and non-surgical treatments.
- Careful patient selection is key in determining a favorable response to the selected treatment modality.
- Certain interventions described in this chapter, such as endobronchial coils and bronchoscopic thermal vapor ablation are irreversible and hence careful discussion and planning is critical prior to their application.

- Pharmacological and non-pharmacological treatment of emphysema should be optimized prior to any surgical or bronchoscopic intervention in order to prevent complications such as infections, pneumonias or coil-associated opacities.

DISCLOSURES

The authors have no disclosures or conflicts of interest.

REFERENCES

1. Brantigan OC, Mueller E. Surgical treatment of pulmonary emphysema. Am Surg 1957;23(9):789–804.
2. Cooper JD, Trulock EP, Triantafillou AN, et al. Bilateral pneumectomy (volume reduction) for chronic obstructive pulmonary disease. J Thorac Card Surg 1995;109(1):106–19.
3. Wakabayashi A, Brenner M, Kayaleh RA, et al. Thoracoscopic carbon dioxide laser treatment of bullous emphysema. Lancet 1991;337:881–3.
4. Wahidi MW, Herth FJF, Chen A, et al. State of the art: interventional pulmonology. Chest 2020;157(3):724–36.
5. Herth FJ, Eberhard R, Gompelmann D, et al. Bronchoscopic lung volume reduction with a dedicated coil: a clinical pilot study. Ther Adv Respir Dis 2010;4(4):225–31.
6. Lador F, Hachulla A-L, Hohn O, et al. Pulmonary perfusion changes as assessed by contrast-enhanced dual-energy computed tomography after endoscopic lung volume reduction by coils. Respiration 2016;92(6):404–13.
7. Sciurba FC, Criner GJ, Strange C, et al. Effect of endobronchial coils vs usual care on exercise tolerance in patients with severe emphysema: the RENEW randomized clinical trial. JAMA 2016;315(20):2178–89.
8. Deslée G, Mal H, Dutau H, et al. Lung volume reduction coil treatment vs. usual care in patients with severe emphysema: The REVOLENS randomized clinical trial. JAMA 2016;315:175–84.
9. Deslée G, Leroy S, Perotin JM, et al. Two-year follow-up after endobronchial coil treatment in emphysema: results from the REVOLENS study. Eur Respir J 2017;50(6):1701740.
10. Garner JL, Kemp SV, Srikanthan K, et al. 5-year survival after endobronchial coil implantation: secondary analysis of the first randomised controlled trial, RESET. Respiration 2020;99:154–62.
11. ClinicalTrials.gov Identifier: NCT03360396. Available at: https://clinicaltrials.gov/ct2/show/NCT03360396.
12. Marchetti N, Kaufman T, Chandra D, et al. Endobronchial coils versus lung volume reduction surgery or medical therapy for treatment of advanced

homogenous emphysema. Chronic Obstr Pulm Dis 2018;5(2):87–96.

13. Dutau H, Bourru D, Guinde J, et al. Successful late removal of endobronchial coils. Chest 2016;150(6): e143–5.

14. Slebos D, ten Hacken N, Hetzel M, et al. Endobronchial coils for endoscopic lung volume reduction: best practice recommendations from an expert panel. Respiration 2018;96(1):1–11.

15. Snell GI, Hopkins P, Westall G, et al. A feasibility and safety study of bronchoscopic thermal vapor ablation: a novel emphysema therapy. Ann Thorac Surg 2009;88(6):1993–8.

16. Gompelmann D, Eberhardt R, Ernst A, et al. The localized inflammatory response to bronchoscopic thermal vapor ablation. Respiration 2013;86:324–31.

17. Herth FJ, Valipour A, Shah PL, et al. Segmental volume reduction using thermal vapour ablation in patients with severe emphysema: 6-month results of the multicentre, parallel-group, open-label, randomised controlled STEP-UP trial. Lancet Respir Med 2016;4(3):185–93.

18. Shah PL, Gompelmann D, Valipour A, et al. Thermal vapour ablation to reduce segmental volume in patients with severe emphysema: STEP-UP 12 month results. Lancet Respir Med 2016;4:e44–5.

19. Gompelmann D, Shah PL, Valipour A, et al. Bronchoscopic thermal vapor ablation: best practice recommendations from an expert panel on endoscopic lung volume reduction. Respiration 2018;1–9. https://doi.org/10.1159/000489815.

20. ClinicalTrials.gov Identifier: NCT03670121. Available at: https://clinicaltrials.gov/ct2/show/NCT03670121.

21. Canning BJ. Reflex regulation of airway smooth muscle tone. J Appl Physiol (1985) 2006;101(3): 971–85.

22. Kistemaker LE, Gosens R. Acetylcholine beyond bronchoconstriction: roles in inflammation and remodeling. Trends Pharmacol Sci 2015;36:164–71.

23. Slebos DJ, Klooster K, Koegelenberg CF, et al. Targeted lung denervation for moderate to severe COPD: a pilot study. Thorax 2015;70:411–9.

24. Kistemaker LE, Slebos DJ, Meurs H, et al. Anti-inflammatory effects of targeted lung denervation in patients with COPD. Eur Respir J 2015;46:1489–92.

25. Refaely Y, Dransfield M, Kramer MR, et al. Biologic lung volume reduction therapy for advanced homogeneous emphysema. Eur Respir J 2010;36(1):20–7.

26. Bakeer M, Abdelgawad TT, El-Metwaly R, et al. Low cost biological lung volume reduction therapy for advanced emphysema. Int J Chron Obstruct Pulmon Dis 2016;11:1793–800.

27. Come CE, Kramer MR, Dransfield MT, et al. A randomised trial of lung sealant versus medical therapy for advanced emphysema. Eur Respir J 2015;46(3):651–62.

28. Shah PL, Slebos D-J, Cardoso PFG, et al. Bronchoscopic lung-volume reduction with Exhale airway stents for emphysema (EASE trial): randomized, sham-controlled, multicentre trial. Lancet 2011; 378(9795):997–1005.

29. Criner GJ, Sue R, Wright S, et al. A multicenter randomized controlled trial of Zephyr endobronchial valve treatment in heterogenous emphysema (LIBERATE). Am J Resp Crit Care Med 2018;198(9):1151–64.

30. Pienta MJ, Zhang P, Derstine BA, et al. Analytic morphomics predict outcomes after lung transplantation. Ann Thorac Surg 2018;105:399–405.

Moving?

Make sure your subscription moves with you!

To notify us of your new address, find your **Clinics Account Number** (located on your mailing label above your name), and contact customer service at:

Email: journalscustomerservice-usa@elsevier.com

800-654-2452 (subscribers in the U.S. & Canada)
314-447-8871 (subscribers outside of the U.S. & Canada)

Fax number: 314-447-8029

Elsevier Health Sciences Division
Subscription Customer Service
3251 Riverport Lane
Maryland Heights, MO 63043

*To ensure uninterrupted delivery of your subscription, please notify us at least 4 weeks in advance of move.

ELSEVIER